英文医学论文写作教程

Writing of English Medical Papers

主　编　陈　战

副主编　韩　涛　李成华　鲍　霞　曲　　悃　孔冉冉　宋红波

编　者　（以姓氏笔画为序）

孔冉冉　曲　悃　刘晓燕　李成华　邱　冬　宋红波

陈　战　陈涵静　周　茜　姚秋慧　徐　丽　韩　涛

鲍　霞

人民卫生出版社

·北　京·

版权所有，侵权必究！

图书在版编目（CIP）数据

英文医学论文写作教程 / 陈战主编 . —北京：人
民卫生出版社，2020.8（2024.1 重印）
ISBN 978-7-117-29674-8

Ⅰ. ①英… Ⅱ. ①陈… Ⅲ. ①医学 – 英语 – 论文 – 写
作 Ⅳ. ①R

中国版本图书馆 CIP 数据核字（2020）第 127223 号

人卫智网	www.ipmph.com	医学教育、学术、考试、健康， 购书智慧智能综合服务平台
人卫官网	www.pmph.com	人卫官方资讯发布平台

英文医学论文写作教程

Yingwen Yixue Lunwen Xiezuo Jiaocheng

主　　编：陈　战
出版发行：人民卫生出版社（中继线 010-59780011）
地　　址：北京市朝阳区潘家园南里 19 号
邮　　编：100021
E - mail：pmph @ pmph.com
购书热线：010-59787592　010-59787584　010-65264830
印　　刷：北京盛通数码印刷有限公司
经　　销：新华书店
开　　本：787×1092　1/16　**印张：**11
字　　数：247 千字
版　　次：2020 年 8 月第 1 版
印　　次：2024 年 1 月第 4 次印刷
标准书号：ISBN 978-7-117-29674-8
定　　价：42.00 元

打击盗版举报电话：010-59787491　E-mail：WQ @ pmph.com
质量问题联系电话：010-59787234　E-mail：zhiliang @ pmph.com

前　　言

随着医药国际交流与合作的不断深入，医学工作者需要将研究成果发表在国际医药期刊上。同时，越来越多的医学院校要求研究生撰写英语论文，提高学术素养，撰写英文医学论文的需求日益增长。但是目前英文医学论文存在写作难、发表慢、数量少、质量低等问题，因此，提高英文医学论文撰写能力是必须的。

本教材是编者在长期教学实践的基础上，结合自身撰写英文医学论文的经验，并参照相关医学论文写作专著编写而成。教材由上、中、下篇组成，共十章。上篇主要介绍学术英语、学术论文和学术不端及规避；中篇是本教材的主体部分，主要介绍英文医学论文写作的步骤和技巧、论文投稿的流程和注意事项、英文医学论文的组成部分（文题、署名与单位、摘要、关键词、引言、材料与方法、结果、讨论、结论、参考文献等）和各部分的写作方法、留学文书的写作方法（个人综述、个人简历和推荐信），各部分从写作方法与技巧的精要介绍入手，结合范文或例句进行点评，介绍常用句型，分析常见误例，并辅以针对性的写作练习；下篇主要介绍英文医学论文写作中的语言运用，分别从词汇层面、语法层面和句法层面介绍论文写作中需要注意的语言现象，并结合误例，分析常见的语言错误，同时还介绍了标点符号的使用及注意事项。书末提供各章的练习答案。

本教材遵循"实用、规范、典型、精炼"的原则，对英文医学论文写作的讲解力求切中要点，深入浅出，列举的范文和范例力求规范、实用，选用的误例力求典型，练习注重对基本写作方法和技巧的训练，以期提高学生英文医学论文写作水平，启发创新思维和创造能力，增强学术素养和学术能力，促进学术交流与知识更新。

本教材内容系统全面，实用性强，既可作为高等医学院校本科生和研究生医学论文写作课程的教材，也可为临床医生和高等医学院校在职人员提高论文写作水平提供参考。

本教材在最新印制的过程中，适逢全党全国深入贯彻落实党的二十大精神之时，党的二十大报告指出："加强教材建设和管理""加快建设高质量教育体系"，为构建高质量医药教材体系指出了方向。编写教材是一项繁重的工作，尽管在编写过程中做了很多努力，但由于经验不足，水平有限，编写过程中可能会存在诸多问题。希望使用者提出宝贵意见，以便不断改进和提高。

编　者

2023 年 7 月

目　录

上篇

学术论文概论

第一章 学术英语

英语大致可以分为通用英语（English for General Purposes，EGP）和专门用途英语（English for Specific Purposes，ESP）两类。学术英语（English for Academic Purposes，EAP）为 ESP 的分支，是基于需求分析开设的与某种特定职业和学科相关的英语。EAP 还可以细分为两类：一是专业学术英语（English for Specific Academic Purposes，ESAP），如医学英语、计算机英语等专业学科英语；二是通用学术英语（English for General Academic Purposes，EGAP），如英语听力技巧、学术写作、文献查阅等各个专业通用的语言知识和技能。

一、国外相关理论研究梳理

1964 年，Halliday、McIntosh 和 Strevens 合著的《语言科学与语言教学》（*The Linguistic Sciences and Language Teaching*）一书提出语域分析（register analysis）的概念，认为通过大量取样特殊人群所使用的语言，进行观察、录音和分析，就有可能设置一门传授这种语言的教学课程。Halliday 等人的观点为 EAP 课程构建提供了理论依据。1969 年，Crystal 和 Davy 出版的《英语语体调查》（*Investigating English Style*）对一系列评论、宗教、报纸报道、法律文书等语域的语言进行了研究，从而开拓了 ESP 和 EAP 研究的重要领域。20 世纪 70 年代，EAP 研究有了显著发展，Huddleston 使用书面科技语言材料进行句法结构的分析；Candlin、Bruton 和 Leather 对医院急救室话语进行分析；美国华盛顿学派的 Trimble 运用语篇分析的方法分析了科技英语语篇。语言学家 Widdowson 认为"在语言教学中，我们没有给作为交流工具的语言足够的和系统的关注……现在我们应把注意力转向专门用途英语研究，特别是科技英语研究"。从语域分析概念的提出，到对某一领域语篇的分析和对 ESP 的重视，作为 ESP 分支的学术英语的地位日渐突出。

二、国内相关理论研究梳理

20 世纪 70 年代末，我国英语教育界才开始关注学术英语教学。1986 年，许国璋就提出"中学学习普通英语，大学学习分科英语，研究生学习专业英语"的"三级英语教学"设想。刘润清指出"将来的英语学习不再是单纯的英语学习，而是与其他学科结合起来，将来的英语教学是越来越多地与某一个方面的专业知识相结合，或者说与另一个学科的知识相结合起来"。

21 世纪初以来，教育主管部门逐步把 EAP 教学摆到更重要的位置。2007 年颁布的《大学英语课程教学要求》将学生的英语能力分为三个层次，分别提出不同要求，即一般要求、较高要求和更高要求。其中"更高要求"的标准是,突出英语能力与专业学习的联系,体现学以致用,要求学生"能听懂用英语讲授的专业课程和英语讲座;能在国际会议和专业交流中宣读论文并参加讨论;能比较顺利地阅读所学专业的英语文献和资料;能用英语撰写所学专业的简短报告和论文;能借助词典翻译所学专业的文献资料"。2015 年,《大学英语教学指南》正式把 EAP 纳入大学英语课程体系。

三、国内外学术英语教学实践

国内外许多高校进行了学术英语教学实践。世界高校的大学英语教学主要是专门用途英语教学,尤其是为学生专业课程服务的学术英语教学,不管是英美等以英语为母语的国家,还是诸如日本、泰国、中国香港等以英语为外语的国家或地区,学术英语课都是一门必修课。日本东京大学和京都大学的大学英语教学一年级为通用学术英语,二至四年级为特殊学术英语。我国香港高校是以学术英语为主,到了高年级有少量和专业或行业相关的特殊学术英语。我国台湾成功大学专门成立了 ESP 教学中心,积极推动专业英语教学。

医学院校也开展了学术英语教学,逐步提高学生的医学人文素养,培养学生在医院场景中进行有效英语交流的能力,指导学生阅读并了解学术语言的特点,学习学术论文的撰写格式和文体特征。

（李成华）

第二章 学术论文

《科学技术报告、学位论文和学术论文的编写格式》(*Presentation of Scientific and Technical Reports, Dissertations and Scientific Papers*)(GB7713-87)明确提出:"学术论文是某一学术课题在实验性、理论性或观测性上具有新的科学研究成果或创新见解和知识的科学记录;或是某种已知原理应用于实际中取得新进展的科学总结,用以提供学术会议上宣读、交流或讨论;或在学术刊物上发表;或作其他用途的书面文件。学术论文应提供新的科技信息,其内容应有所发现、有所发明、有所创造、有所前进,而不是重复、模仿、抄袭前人的工作。"在社会科学领域,人们通常把表达科研成果的论文称为学术论文。简而言之,学术论文是指对某一领域的某个问题,通过某种方法进行科学的探索和思考而写成的以论述为主的文章,是科学研究成果的文字表述。

一、学术论文的特点

与普通论文不同,学术论文有自身的特点,主要体现为:学术性、科学性、创新性和理论性。

(一) 学术性

所谓学术性,是指研究探讨的内容具有专门性和系统性,即是以科学领域里某一专业性问题作为研究对象。当然,有些学术论文是不同专业人员共同研究的成果。

首先,从内容上看,学术论文有明显的专业性,是作者运用系统的专业知识去论证和解决专业性很强的学术问题。内容的专业性是学术论文区别于一般文章的最重要标志。其次,从语言表达看,学术论文是运用专业术语和专业性图表、符号来表达内容的,阅读对象是同行。因此,需要把学术问题表达得简洁、准确、规范,专业术语使用很多。

(二) 科学性

所谓科学性,就是指研究探讨的内容准确、思维严密、推理合乎逻辑。

首先是研究态度的科学性。从事社会科学研究,就必须从大量的材料出发,通过分析材料得出结论;从事实验研究,就应该对课题进行系统实验,从大量的实验数据中分析,综合得出结论。其次是研究方法的科学性。要把握好习近平新时代中国特色社会主义思想的世界观和方法论,坚持好、运用好贯穿其中的立场、观点、方法,对某一研究对象进行科学探讨。先用归纳法,再用演绎法,从大量的具体材料去归纳,从个别到一般,以归纳为基础,再做分析,最后得出结论。再次是内容和观点的科学性,这就要求论文论点正确、概念明确、论据充分、推理严密、语言准确。观点是学术研究的成果结论,这个结论须反映客观事物的本质规律和客观真理,经得起推敲和逻辑推理。

(三)创新性

创新是科技发展的第一动力。因此,创新性是学术论文的特点之一。论文的创新可以是研究内容的创新,也可以是研究方法和研究结论的创新。主要表现在以下几个方面:

- 填补空白的新发现、新发明、新理论;
- 对原有理论在继承基础上的发展、创新、完善;
- 在众说纷纭中提出独立见解;
- 推翻前人在某一研究领域的定论;
- 运用新的方法对现有资料进行创造性地加工;
- 对前人鲜有涉猎的内容进行研究。

(四)理论性

所谓理论性,是指论文作者思维的理论性、论文结论的理论性和论文表达的论证性。

思维的理论性,即研究者对研究对象的思考,不是停留在零散的感性认识上,而是运用概念、判断、分析、归纳、推理等思辨的方法,深刻认识研究对象的本质和规律,经过高度概括和升华,使之成为理论。结论的理论性,即学术论文的结论是建立在充分的事实归纳基础上,通过理性思维,高度概括其本质和规律,使之升华为理论,理性思维水平越高,结论的理论价值就越高。表达的论证性,即对结论展开逻辑的、精密的论证,从而具有说服力。

二、学术论文的类型

按照不同的划分标准,学术论文可分为不同类型。按研究领域分,学术论文可分为自然科学论文和社会科学论文;按研究内容分,可分为理论研究论文和应用研究论文;根据研究方法,可分为图书馆研究和实验研究;按性质和功能分,可分为论说性论文、综述性论文、评论性论文和驳论性论文。论说性论文是用大量事实、数据和材料,从正面阐释,论证自己的观点;综述性论文是对某一时期、某一领域、某一学科的研究进展进行概括和梳理,分析现状,指出存在问题,明确发展方向,提出研究建议;评论性论文是对某一学术成果、期刊论文或专著的内容和观点进行评估、鉴定,指出其成就,分析其价值,指出其中的问题与不足,书评属于此类;驳论性论文是反驳对方提出的观点,提出自己的见解,商榷类文章属于此类。

三、学术论文的组成

撰写学术论文,尤其是科技论文,需要遵循一定的规范,一般包括开篇(preface)、主体(IMRaD)和收尾(end)三个部分。

开篇 包括标题/文题(title)、作者(author)、摘要(abstract)和关键词(keywords)。

主体 称作"IMRaD Format",包括 introduction、methods、results、discussion 等部分。

收尾 包括致谢(acknowledgement)、参考文献(reference)和附件(supplementary material)。

法国化学家和生物学家巴斯德(Louis Pasteur)19 世纪 70 年代首次采用 IMRaD 格式发表生物医学科技论文。1972 年,美国国家标准化研究所建立了 IMRaD 格式作为报告科学信息的规范。20 世纪初,学界逐渐形成 IMRaD 论文格式。

《柳叶刀》撰稿编辑 Sharp 简明扼要地将这种模式定义为"以引言开始,跟随以方法,然后是结果,最后是讨论的顺序,称为 IMRaD 格式。"(The sequence of having an introduction followed by the methodology,then the results and lastly the discussion.)IMRaD 是 introduction,methods,results 和 discussion 四个英文单词的首字母缩略。这一模式不仅适用于自然科学,也适用于社会科学学术论文。

瑞典皇家技术学院 Johansson 列出了 IMRaD 包含的主要内容:

The **INTRODUCTION** section normally contains:① nature and scope of the problem（What is the problem and why is it important to study?）,② literature review（What has already been done?）,③ methods（What methods have been used and why?）,④ results and ⑤ conclusions.

The **METHODS** section should give full details of data collection,experimental design,sampling techniques,and so on. In a case study,it is important to elaborate on rationale for selection of the case to study. In the natural sciences,this is often called **material and method**. In the social sciences,it is common to introduce a section called **theory and method**,sometimes divided in two sections:**theoretical framework and method**.

In the **RESULTS** section the reader is told what your findings were. It is not enough to present your findings in a table or a graph;you need to interpret them for your reader. Figures and tables must be numbered and labeled and referred to in the text.

The **DISCUSSION/CONCLUSION** section should discuss the results,not recapitulate them. But there is normally a short summary of the main results. Discuss principles,relationships,and generalizations shown by the results.

The main body of the section is normally organized according to some kind of logical system,for instance,past-to-present,general-to-specific,theoretical-to-practical. The discussion might be written in a more personal manner than the rest of the report. It could contain reflections on the learning process and shortcomings of the inquiry. It is also a good idea to mention possible future work.

四、学术论文的语体风格

学术论文在用词、句法、修辞等方面有其自身特点。一般说来,学术英语具有客观性、正式性、复杂性、明晰性、模糊性、被动性等特点。

(一) 客观性(Objectivity)

学术论文不同于一般文体文章,它强调学术观点的阐释和信息的表达。因此,学术论文应避免使用带有感情色彩的表达,使用中性的、无偏见的、客观的表述。如我们常使用这样的句式:

From the above analysis,it can be inferred that...

The above analysis seems to indicate that...

According to the above analysis, ...

The data indicate that...

试比较:

（1）It is a very interesting and practical study.

　　In my opinion, it is a very interesting and practical study.

（2）It is not easy to conclude what life might be 5,000 years ago without the intervention of medicine.

　　I think it is not easy to conclude what life might be 5,000 years ago without the intervention of medicine.

（二）正式性（Formality）

学术论文相对比较正式，因此在写作中较多地使用第三人称主语、复杂词语、完整句式、书面语、相关领域的专业词汇等，而不能使用俚语、缩略形式、口语表达、省略句等，宾语从句中的 that 通常也不能省略。学科术语的表达尽量规范化，不要随意化。

试比较:

（1）It is concluded that...

　　It's concluded that...

（2）Numerous specialists maintain/state that...

　　Some experts think that...

（3）Therefore, .../Thus...

　　So, ...

试比较:

Casual Voice（口语）	Consultative Voice（一般书面语）	Academic Voice（学术用语）
Hey, dude, no way you can sit here!	You are not allowed to sit in this area, because it is a safety concern.	This area must be kept clear for foot traffic.
Yuck! I hate broccoli with those nasty, stinking mushrooms. Why do we gotta have these things again, man?	I'd prefer not to have this particular vegetable again, if it's possible. Does anyone really enjoy this combination of mushrooms and broccoli?	Very few people enjoy this broccoli and mushroom dish. Therefore, it will not be served again within this calendar year, or the servers will be killed.
Sweet! I love those Indiana Jones movies! They're awesome with the whip and the bugs and stuff. Everyone loves those flicks!	Indiana Jones films are really very popular with your age group. Critics can't decide why such an old character is so appealing.	Hollywood is perplexed at the reasons that Indiana Jones is so favored by such young audiences. The answer remains a mystery.

（三）复杂性（Complexity）

学术语言是一种书面语言，在词汇、句法、语法层面，都比口语复杂得多。主要表现为：词语较长，多用名词结构，用词变化多；句式复杂，常有从句；时态多变，不局限于现在时态，被动语态较多。Halliday 在《口语和书面语》一书中专门做了比较：

Spoken：You can control the trains this way and if you do that you can be quite sure that they'll be able to run more safely and more quickly than they would otherwise，no matter how bad the weather is.

Written：The use of this method of control unquestionably leads to safer and faster train running in the most adverse weather conditions.

两者的差异还体现在语法、用词、人称等方面。

试比较：

Spoken	Written
Whenever I'd visited there before，I'd ended up feeling that it would be futile if I tried to do anything more.	Every previous visit had left me with a sense of the futility of further action on my part.
The cities in Switzerland had once been peaceful，but they changed when people became violent.	Violence changed the face of once peaceful Swiss cities.
Because the technology has improved it's less risky than it used to be when you install them at the same time，and it doesn't cost so much either.	Improvements in technology have reduced the risk and high costs associated with simultaneous installation.
The people in the colony rejoiced when it was promised that things would change in this way.	Opinion in the colony greeted the promised change with enthusiasm.

（四）明晰性（Explicitness）

学术论文的明晰性主要体现在：

学术观点及其组织形式要明确。如写作思路、观点陈述的改变要有明确的词来表达，如 however、furthermore、nonetheless 等。

观点相似或相悖要明确。如两位研究者观点相似，可用 similarly、the same is also true of 等，如观点不同，可用 in contrast 等。

举例说明要明确。如举例子时，可使用 for example、for instance 等。

引用说明要明确。如引用别人的观点或文字表述，应明确标出。

（五）模糊性（Hedging）

学术论文的模糊性，不是指语言文字表达不清楚、含糊，而是说话要留有余地，不要说得太满，亦即话语谨慎，不要武断地下结论。避免使用过度概括的词语，如 always，every，改用 often、many/much 等；使用模糊限制语，如 probably、seems、might be、tend to、indicate、the majority of、there is a tendency for、it would seem that 等表述。学术论文的模糊性主要体现在结论部分。常用词汇、句式如：

动词：seem，tend，appear，indicate，suggest

副词：sometimes，often，usually

句式：It could be the case that...

　　　It might be suggested that...

It appears that...

This suggests that...

（六）被动性（Passiveness）

学术论文常使用被动语态客观地描述材料方法或表达观点，其被动性主要体现在材料方法和结论部分。如：

Randomized controlled trials were included while quasi-randomized controlled trials were not.

Multiple publications reporting the same groups of participants were excluded to reduce overlapping data.

那么，学术论文中能否使用第一人称 we、I 作主语？一般认为，可以使用 we 指称自己的研究团队。表达"人们"或者"某人认为"的时候，则通常使用被动语态。如：

We compared the outcomes between the study protocol and the final published trial.

It is all known that cardiac Purkinje cells played a crucial role in the propagation of impulse from atrioventricular node to ventricular muscle and may initiate a variety of ventricular arrhythmias.

强调作者的观点、论文的写作目的、实验的方法等，可以使用如下句式：

This article describes an algorithm for clustering sequences into index classes.

The present paper presents a set of criteria for selecting such a component.

This review aims to clarify the classification of toxicity in TCM.

（李成华）

第三章 学术不端及规避

学术不端（plagiarism），又称抄袭、剽窃。《现代汉语词典》把抄袭定义为："照着别人的作品、作业等写下来当作自己的"。《朗文当代高级英语辞典》把 plagiarism 定义为："an idea, phrase, or story that has been copied from another person's work, without stating where it came from"。由此可见，英汉语中对"抄袭"的界定相似，这种抄袭发生在学术论文中，就是学术不端。

一、学术不端（Plagiarism）

美国现代语言联合会编写的《论文作者手册》指出："剽窃是在你的写作中使用他人的观点或表述而没有恰当地注明出处……这包括逐字复述、复制他人的写作，或使用不属于你自己的观点而没有给出恰当的引用……对论文而言，剽窃有两种：**一种是剽窃观点**，用了别人的观点而不注明，让人误以为是自己的观点；**一种是剽窃文字**，照抄别人的文字表述而没有注明出处且未用引号，让人误以为是你自己的表述。当然，由于论文注重观点的原创性，前者要比后者严重。而普及性的文章却不同，因为并不注重观点的原创性，所以不要求对来自别人的观点一一注明，因此只看重文字表述是否剽窃。"

当然，修改语法表达、增加个别词语或改变主动、被动语态而未注明出处的，也是抄袭。经文献检测系统发现论文内容（包括图、表）的重复率大于 30%，不管是否注明参考文献、来源出处和解释说明（包括未经原文作者的同意和授权的编译、翻译论文，也不管作者是有意的或无意的），即可认定为抄袭。简而言之，在论文中不正确的引用就是抄袭。

二、引证（Citation/Quotation）

所谓引证，就是引用事实或言论、著作作为根据。在科学论文中，引证就是引用别人的观点、方法、结果和结论，并必须注明出处。

人文社科类论文在引经据典或引用权威人士的讲话或论断时，需一字不差，因此需要引号引出。科技论文中的引用是必需的，因此论文末尾附有参考文献。科技论文重点引用观点、方法或结论，不需要整段引用，因此不必使用引号。但这并不意味着科技论文中的引用不能用引号，如果一字不差地引用观点，也应用引号引出，同时标注在参考文献中。这既是对原作者的尊重，也是基本的学术规范。

三、改写（Paraphrase）

剽窃不仅仅指抄袭文字。如果参照别人在论文或著作中已经发表的观点进行改写，也应当致谢作者,列在参考文献中,否则亦视为剽窃。

四、避免学术不端

1. 从阅读中总结提炼,用自己的话表达观点。

2. 若必须引用,须注意:

(1)正确对待引用。不必担心引用过多,引用文献在一定程度上表明作者对某一话题的熟悉程度;也不必担心引用过少,但要确保引用最权威、最新的研究资料。

(2)区别直接引用和间接引用。直接引用作者的表述时,应用引号标明,并列在参考文献中;引用观点不用引号标明,但须列在参考文献中。

(3)引用有价值的观点。注意引用行业专家的观点,有引用有评论。

（李成华）

中篇
英文医学论文写作

第一章　医学科研论文的写作步骤与技巧

医学论文是医学科学研究和工作的书面总结,是开展经验交流和提高学术水平的重要工具,其目的在于阐明作者的新发现、新方法、新经验或新观点。把科学研究结果撰写成学术论文并成功发表,不仅要广泛收集、精心整理和科学地分析资料,而且还要掌握撰写医学论文的方法和技巧,提高论文质量。

第一节　论文文题的选择与确定

论文选题是撰写学术研究论文的开端,是至关重要而又艰难的第一步,一个好的选题可以说是成功的一半。

一、选题的原则

论文选题应该遵守以下四个基本原则:创新、可行、需求、协作。

1. 贵在创新　论文贵在守正创新,要不断推进实践基础上的理论创新。论文的创新表现在:文题新、内容新、方法新、观点新。创新性又叫先进性,是科研论文的精髓,决定论文的生命。无论是创新性还是先进性,基本点就是要体现在"新"上。科技论文不同于一般教材,教材叙述的内容一般是比较成型或定性的东西,而论文是最新研究成果的反映或新获得经验的总结,也就是说,必须具有区别于前人或其他人的独到之处。还需指出,要想使自己的论文在审查时不被编辑或审稿人退稿,最好不要让自己的文章与文末的参考文献同名。

2. 实际可行　撰写论文需要量力而行,要有充实的素材作基础。因此,选题要选自己最熟悉、最感兴趣的东西,而且是力所能及的。只有这样,根据手头掌握的材料才有可能写出好的文章来。

3. 符合需求　选题要为民之所需,应聚焦实践中遇到的新问题、改革发展稳定存在的深层次问题、人民群众急愁难盼的问题、生物医学领域中未被人类认识的重大问题。在日常工作中遇到的各种需要研究解决的问题,都可以作为选题的参考。

4. 多方协作　现代的科研绝非凭一己之力所能及,需要多学科、多专业、跨单位、跨地区的协作才能开展,有些课题甚至必须由国际合作来完成。同样,写作选题的确定也需集思广益,反复推敲。数据的完整、统计学处理及参考文献的获取,都需要多人、多单位的协作。

简而言之,选题最重要的是创新和求实。创新是指尽量选择本专业及其交叉学科前沿领域中他人未曾开展或者值得改进的课题。求实包含两层含义,选题既要满足生产活动的客观需要,又要量力而行,难度适当。

二、文题的要求

文题主要体现文章的中心内容,是论文主要内容和中心思想的高度概括。一个好的的文题,既要言简意赅又要信息丰富,要尽可能用较少的文字概括全文的中心内容。医学科研论文的文题要如实反映论文的性质、研究对象和主要观测项目。同时,还需具备可读性、特异性和可检索性。文题独树一帜能够吸引读者,反之,含混不清、没有特色的文题常被读者跳过,尽管该文题可能蕴含重要的内容。

文题应该准确、鲜明、生动、简洁、通俗,能吸引读者阅读,但不同性质的文章对文题有不同的要求。一篇论文往往可以设想几个文题,根据内容进行比较选择,使之既不要过于概括,以致流于空泛、一般化,也不能太繁琐,无法给人留下鲜明的印象。文题过于繁琐,既难以记忆,也给引证带来麻烦。

总之,文题既要言简意赅、高度概括,又要突出新意、反映主题。

三、选题的禁忌

选题要尽量避免以下几种情况:

(1) 有关选题的文献参考资料太少,或者有关资料太多;

(2) 选题所涉及的文献资料内容太难;

(3) 选题本身太倾向于主观判断或个人好恶;

(4) 选题不具备可争议性。

(陈战)

第二节 资料的收集与整理

要想写出高质量的医学论文,不但要具备扎实的专业基础知识,还要了解本专业的新知识和新进展。科学发展是人类长期实践积累的结果,既需要自己积累丰富的知识与经验,也要注意学习和汲取他人的实践经验。因此,在论文撰写前,除精心整理、分析已有资料外,还要大量地查阅医学文献,收集相关信息,积累专业知识。

一、资料收集的内容

收集论文需要的文献资料时,应特别注意收集以下几方面的内容:

(1) 在方法上沿用前人的,或在前人的基础上加以改进的;

(2) 在理论认识上支持本文观点的;

(3) 前人研究的结论与自己文章所述不同,需要加以说明的;

(4) 前人对本文所研究的问题存在争议和正在探讨的。

将这些资料搜集好后,编好序号,以备撰写文章时使用。

二、资料收集的方法

1. 查阅医学论文　有计划地去查阅他人的医学专业论文,特别是结合医学工作中的实际问题去阅读论文,能够大大提高自身的专业理论水平,为日后撰写论文打下扎实基础。

2. 多看医学综述　综述大都是作者收集了大量文献经过分析综合整理而成,内容丰富,包含了某专题的大量信息。通过阅读综述,不仅对某一专题有较全面和深入的了解,而且还可以追踪所引用的文献,查出更多的资料,采取滚雪球的办法掌握某个专题的丰富资料。

3. 阅读教科书和专著　教科书或专著的内容一般是较为系统和成熟的理论,比一般的期刊资料更具权威性,对工作的指导意义更强。因此,阅读教科书和专著可以很好地巩固专业知识和更新知识储备。

4. 做好实验记录　实验一开始就要及时、详细地记录,并随时整理,从中提炼相关结果(数据、现象、照片以及偶然的发现),分段地进行小结与回顾,以便及时发现问题,随时纠正或补充,待实验或临床观察结束,及时进行总结。

三、文献的选取

选取参考文献时,要遵循以下几个要求:

1. 新颖性　文献应以近 3~5 年为主;宜多选刊,少选书,而且是亲自阅读过的原始论文。

2. 代表性　一般而言,中外文献都应该有,不能为显示外语水平或"臆想"的先进性而只选取外文文献,不选取中文文献,更不能因为阅读困难而只选中文文献。国外的不一定都是先进的,但没有又太局限;不选国内的也不全面,国内患者、病种多,研究更多,而且来自国人的诊断结果更符合国情。另一方面,对国外来说,反映中国特色的内容就是新东西。

3. 权威性　选取的文献应是正式发表的;如果有多篇类似文献,一般选择作者知名度高的。

四、资料的整理

资料整理包括审核资料、资料分组、制定整理表格、统计分析等步骤。

1. 审核资料　资料搜集之后应该及时审核,以便随时复查修正。审核的内容主要包括:资料的正确性,如内容是否合乎要求、相关项目是否矛盾、分数与总数是否相等;资料的完整性,如表格数据是否错栏或错行,计量单位是否准确。搜集资料时,应根据论文的需要,把与科研课题有密切关系并要引用的资料保存下来,并注明文献的出处,包括作者、题目、杂志名称、年代、卷、期、起止页码等,漏一不可。

2. 资料分组　分组是根据性质或数量特征把全部资料分为若干组,以反映事物的特征,便于后期论文写作中使用。科学的分组是统计处理的基础,只有在同质的基础上进行分组,才能得出正确的结论。分组太粗或组数太少常常会掩盖资料的信息。

3. 制定整理表格　整理表格主要用于整理和归类原始资料,是提供分析资料的过渡性表格。表格是否直接用于论文,使用表格、图表还是文字描述,取决于哪种形式更易于读者理解,又节省版面。

4. 统计分析　统计的数据,如果未经统计学处理,并不可靠,没有说服力。因此,初稿完成后,凡涉及数据处理的须请统计学专家把关。

上述准备工作完成以后,要根据有关文献资料和实验观察所得的资料,重新核对实验设计中所包含的思想,运用辩证唯物主义的观点,分析设计中哪些观点在理论上成立,而且在实验中得到证实;哪些观点在实验中没有得到证实或未完全证实,需要修改;哪些现象和指标超出原来设想,而且可能有新的启示,需要进行新的分析。通过对实验材料的分析,提炼出能够说明的观点和得到的结果,提出结论,使实验材料和理论认识充分结合起来。以上的准备工作,可以使理论和实践相统一,从而提高论文的水平。

（陈战）

第三节　文　献　检　索

《文献著录总则》(GB3792.1-83)将文献定义为"记录有知识的一切载体"。按照载体的不同,文献可以划分为印刷型、电子型和声像型等。按出版类型,文献可以分为图书、期刊、会议文献、学位论文、科技报告和专利文献等。医学论文写作的各个阶段,无论是确立选题、选择研究方法,还是分析试验数据、撰写结论,都离不开专业而全面的文献检索工作。

文献检索是指根据用户的需求利用检索工具或检索系统查找出符合用户特定需求信息的过程。医学文献检索是指根据学习和工作的需要获取医学相关文献的过程。随着现代网络技术的发展,医学文献检索更多地通过计算机来完成。

一、医学文献检索工具

检索工具是用于报道、存储和查找文献线索的工具和设备的总称,具有报道文献、存储文献、检索文献等基本功能。检索工具按照不同的标准可以划分为不同的种类。医学研究者应根据研究的范围和要求,选择恰当的检索工具。

（一）常用医学检索数据库

1. 中国期刊全文数据库　网址为 http://www.cnki.net,是中国知识基础设施工程(CNKI)的重要组成部分,是由清华大学发起、同方知网产业集团承建的国家重要项目,目前收录国内 9 100 多种综合期刊与专业特色期刊全文,内容覆盖自然科学、工程技术、农业、哲学、医学、人文社会科学等各个领域。其中,中国医院知识总库(CHKD)为医药卫生系统专业人员及其他广大用户提供更新速度快、信息权威性高、命中精准且全面的知识服务,能进行中外文跨库检索及分析、外文单库主题检索、新出版来源导航、网络首发及 HTML 阅读等。

2. 万方医学网　网址为 http://www.wanfangdata.com.cn,是万方数据联合国内医学权威机构、医学期刊编辑部、权威医学专家推出的,面向广大医院、医学院校、科研机构及医疗卫生从业人员的医学信息整合服务、医学知识链接全开放平台,为用户提供期刊杂志、学位论文、会议论文、科技成果等信息检索功能,并提供在线支持服务。

3. **中国生物医学文献数据库(CBM)**　网址为 http://www.sinomed.ac.cn,是中国医学科学院医学信息研究所开发研制的综合性医学文献检索数据库。CBM 收录了 1978 年以来的 1 800 余种中国生物医学期刊,以及汇编、会议论文文献题录 540 余万篇,是目前国内文献收录量最大,涵盖学科门类最全,功能最完善的医学文献数据库之一,是检索中文医学文献的首选数据库。

4. **PubMed**　网址为 http://www.ncbi.nlm.nih.gov/,是国际权威的生物医学文献书目型数据库,是由美国国立医学图书馆所属的国家生物技术信息中心(NCBI)开发的免费互联网生物医学文献数据库。文献主要源自 Medline、Premedline、出版商提供的文献数据库和 NCBI 其他数据库的相关记录等方面。PubMed 具有收录文献范围广、内容覆盖全、检索途径多、检索功能完善、数据更新快等特点。灵活应用 PubMed 的检索限定、临床查询、引文匹配等工具,能大大提高检索效率。PubMed 可以作为检索英文医学文献的首选。

5. **Embase 数据库**　网址为 http://www.embase.com,是由荷兰 Elsevier Science 出版公司建立的书目型数据库,是全球生命科学领域最重要的文献检索工具之一。该数据库在提供丰富的生物医学文献的同时,还广泛地收录药学文献。目前 Embase 中 50% 的记录已经实现与 ScienceDirect,SpringerLink,Cell Press 以及 KARGER 等电子期刊全文数据库的链接,可以方便地获取全文。

6. **谷歌学术搜索及数据库**　网址为 http://scolar.google.com,可以免费搜索各种学术文献,包括期刊论文、学位论文、书籍、预印本、文摘和技术报告等,内容涵盖自然科学、人文科学、社会科学等多种学科。

7. **中国中医药数据库**　网址为 http://cintmed.cintcm.com/cintmed/main.html,是由中国中医科学院研制的中国最大、最权威的中医药专业数据库。其中的中医药学文献分析检索系统和中英文针灸文献分析和检索系统也收录大量中医药文献和针灸文献。

(二)常用医学参考工具书

1. **百科全书**　百科全书是对人类现有知识的编排、浓缩整理和条理化概要记述,具有全面性、系统性和可靠性的特点。常用的中文医学百科全书有《中国大百科全书:中国传统医学》《中国医学百科全书》。

2. **年鉴**　年鉴是按年度系统汇集国内外重大事件、新进展、新知识和新资料,供读者查阅的工具书。一般以当年为限,逐年编辑,常被称为“微型百科全书”。常用的医学类年鉴有《中国卫生年鉴》《中国医药年鉴》《中国内科年鉴》《中国外科年鉴》《中国药学年鉴》等。

3. **手册**　手册是以简明、缩写方式汇集特定领域的文献、资料、信息及有关专业知识的工具书,可分为综合性和专科性两种。常用医学手册有《默克诊疗手册》《临床生化指标参考手册》等。

4. **名录**　名录是提供人物和机构的简明信息的工具书。常用的医学名录有《世界医学院校名录》《中国中医名人榜》《国际医学名人录》等。

5. **词典**　词典是以说明词语的概念、意义和用法为主的工具书。常用的医学词典有 *Dorland's Illustrated Medical Dictionary*（《道兰氏插图医学词典》）、《医学综合征词典》（*Dictionary of Medical Syndromes*）、《诊断学大辞典》、《中药大辞典》等。

6. **图录和表谱**　图录是以图像揭示事物的工具书，表谱是以编年或表格形式记载事物发展的工具书。二者大多按时间顺序编排，主要用于查检时间、历史事件、人物信息等。常用的医药图谱有《针灸穴位解剖图谱》《神经系统 MR 诊断图谱》《全国中草药汇编彩色图谱》《普通外科手术图谱》等。

（三）检索工具书

1. **目录**　也称书目，是将一批相关图书或其他类型的出版物按一定次序编排而成的一种检索工具。图书目录，如《全国新书目》和《全国总书目》，是检索我国出版图书的主要检索工具。期刊目录，如《中文科技资料目录：医药卫生》，收集国内医学及与医学相关的期刊、图书、汇编（内部资料）、学术会议等文献，是查阅国内医学文献的重要检索工具。《国外科技资料目录：医药卫生》是国内出版的检索国外科技文献的刊物，收编了英、法、德、日、俄等语种的医学期刊。

2. **索引**　索引指将书籍和报刊所载的具有检索意义的文章篇名、著者、主题、人名、地名、名词术语等摘录出来，按照一定次序编排成简短的条目，并注明出处、时间、所在文献的页码和文献号等，以供检索的工具书。它提供了查找资料的线索和途径。较常见的索引有《全国报刊索引》《报刊资料索引》*Index Medicus*（IM，《医学索引》）、*Science Citation Index*（SCI，《科学引文索引》）等。

3. **文摘**　文摘是文献内容的浓缩，能简明确切地反映文献内容。将大量文献的文摘配上相应的文献题录，按一定的方法编排而成的检索工具，称为文摘型检索工具，简称为文摘。常用的医学文献文摘有《中国医学文摘》*Excepta Medica*（EM，《医学文摘》）、*Biological Abstracts*（BA，《生物文摘》）和 *Chemical Abstracts*（CA，《化学文摘》）等。

二、医学文献检索途径

文献检索途径指利用文献信息的特征查找文献的方法或渠道。根据外部特征，医学文献检索主要有文献名、著者、序号等途径。

1. **文献名**　文献名途径根据书名、刊名、篇名、特种文献名所编成的索引和目录来查找文献。该途径是在文献名称已知的前提下进行的，适用于某一文献名称的专指性检索，因此具有直接、便捷等优点。

2. **著者**　著者途径以著者姓名为检索标识进行文献检索。著者包括作者、编者、译者等个人、团体、学术会议主办单位等。该途径是在著者已知的前提下利用著者姓名进行检索，可以查阅到同一著者的一批同类或相关的文献资料，因此具有延伸性的特点，但使用该途径检索文献信息时需要注意文种不同和姓名排列方式的差异。

3. **序号**　序号途径以文献出版时所编号码顺序来检索文献。序号包括文献报告号、专利号、国际标准号、文摘号等。由于文献序号具有唯一性的特点,因此该途径可以精准地查找到相应的文献。

三、医学文献检索步骤

文献检索是一个有目的、有计划的信息收集过程。一般来说,医学文献检索遵循以下步骤:

1. 分析检索课题　研究者首先应该分析研究对象,明确文献检索的主题、类别和来源,确定研究内容的文献检索标识,如关键词、作者、作者单位、文献分类号、主题词等,提出具体的检索任务。

2. 选择检索工具　在明确检索任务的基础上,选择相应的检索工具,根据主题要求确定使用印刷型检索或计算机检索。

3. 确定检索方法和检索途径　根据文献类型、语种、收录时间等选择检索方法和途径。

4. 检索并获取文献　研究者可根据新的线索及时调整检索方案和检索工具,补充新的检索标识或采用个性化的途径。最终通过馆藏、馆际互借、向著者索取原文,或通过网上全文传递服务、网上全文数据库、网上出版社等方式获取文献。

(孔冉冉)

第四节　撰写初稿

一、内容构思

构思是撰写论文的准备,也是开始。它是作者对文章整体布局、论点以及依据进行阐明、安排和设计的过程。其内容包括:文章的布局、顺序、层次、段落、内容、观点、材料、怎样开头和结尾。

构思是写文章不可缺少的准备过程,构思时文章的主题中心要明确,用以表现的材料要充分、典型、新颖,结构上要严谨、环环相扣。只有潜心构思,才能思路流畅,写好提纲和文章。

二、拟定提纲

提纲是论文的基本骨架,有了提纲,作者写起来才会目标明确,思路开通。拟定提纲,一方面可帮助作者从全局着眼,明确层次和重点,使文章写得有条理,结构严谨;另一方面,通过提纲把作者的构思、观点用文字固定下来,做到目标明确,主次分明。随着思路的进一步深化,会逐渐发现新问题、新方法和新观点,不断地修改和完善原来的构思。

提纲是论文的轮廓,应尽量写得详细一些。提纲的拟写多采用标题式。

标题式提纲以简明的标题形式把文章的内容概括出来,用最简明的词语标示出某部分或某段落的主要内容。这样既简明扼要,又便于记忆,是医学科研工作者常用的写作方法。例如,实验研究型论文提纲通常使用以下结构:

文题:……

1. 引言

　①课题的提出

　②研究的目的

2. 材料与方法

　①实验目的、原理、条件、仪器和试剂

　②实验方法:分组情况,观察指标,记录方法

　③操作过程

　④出现的问题和采取的对策

3. 结果与分析

　①结果

　②统计学处理

　③结果的可信度

　④再现性

4. 讨论(结论)

5. 参考文献

提纲的作用在于启发写作的积极性和创造性。在实际的写作过程中,作者应做到既有纲可循,又不拘泥于提纲,尽可能地拓宽思路,才能写出好的论文。

三、撰写初稿的要求和技巧

(一) 写作要求

1. 内容完整,数据齐备　要将事先想到并认为需要写进论文的内容全部写进去,多了删减容易,少了补充困难。数据,尤其是说明结论的结果数据,更是缺一不可。

2. 用词达意,杜绝歧义　用词达意首先是保证科学术语的规范化。例如,过去的"白血球"现规范为"白细胞","过敏反应"规范为"变态反应"。这种改变一经确定,个人便不能随意换用,不存在"修辞"问题,没有随意性。

除了专业术语外,其他词语的适当变化还是必要的。例如,"因为"可以变换为"由于""所以""因此";"产品购自……"可以变换为"为……的产品""由……生产/提供";"显示"可以变换为"表明""提示""证明""揭示"。

其次,词义要确切,表达要严谨,避免前后矛盾或者歧义。例如,"本组 41 例患者,女性23 例,男性 18 例,男女比例为 1.3：1。"稍加琢磨,这句话前后表述存在矛盾。前面的表述是女性比男性多,可后面的表达是"男女比例为 1.3：1",意思应该是男性多,女性少。综合整句的意思,应该把"男女比例"改成"女性与男性之比",或者改成"男性 18 例,女性 23 例,男女比例为 1：1.3"。

3. 语言精炼,缩写规范

（1）语言精炼:高水平的论文除了内容的先进性、科学性,写作上应力求做到以最小的篇幅容纳最大量的信息,因此必须摒弃冗句赘词。只有精炼的语言,才能赢得众多的读者。

（2）缩写规范:采用缩略语可以精炼文字,减少篇幅,节省版面。例如:computed/computerized tomography（计算机 X 线断层照相术）→ CT,magnetic resonance imaging（磁共振成像）→ MRI。另外,缩略语便于阅读和记忆。例如,publication of medicine → PubMed。

4. 突出新意,结论得当　俗话说,文贵在新。但是,作者在全力展示论文新意的时候,不能言过其实。任何夸大其词都会引起审稿人和读者的反感和不信任,进而导致退稿。结论得当是指得出的结论具体可估,"结果理想"或"疗效满意"之类的结论就不足取。

（二）写作技巧

1. 顺序写作,一气呵成　如果对拟写内容、形式及结构已经非常清楚,则可顺着思路,一鼓作气完成初稿。这时不必追求语言修辞、结构紧凑、层次清晰、逻辑顺畅等,这些工作可以在后期修改时完成。只要资料或素材完整,提纲合理,一气呵成完成论文初稿并非难事。

2. 分段写作,随时补充　撰写论文并非每个人都能一气呵成,写作中常常会感到无从下笔,不是对运用的语言不满意,就是逻辑不顺,段落搭配不和谐。遇到这种情况,不妨留出空白,做上记号,后期再斟酌完善。在细节上花费太多心思,往往容易打乱思路,影响全文的整体思考和组织。

3. 讨论与参考文献　讨论是医学科研论文难写的部分,也是写作水平的主要体现之处。以论文内容为依据,进行分析、比较,写出结果的原因,表明观点,提出见解,突显论文或研究成果的特色,并指出存在的问题,展望相关领域前景。注意评价成果要做到实事求是,不能言过其实。

参考文献的引用好坏,不是以引用的多少为标准,而是看引用得准不准,而且要选取最具权威性、代表性和针对性的文献。

4. 论文摘要的写作　摘要是从论文中摘录出来的要点,是概括而不加注释或评论的简短陈述,应简练、准确、完整而能独立成文,可以作为独立的资料来使用和保存。摘要的特点是短、精、完整。短,因容量限制;精,即集中体现文章的精华,反映全文的信息量;完整,指摘要是全文的高度浓缩,能独立成章,本身就能成为一篇完整的短文,具有与文章同等的阅读、储存、评价和使用价值。

（陈战）

第五节　修 改 初 稿

修改是论文写作中不可缺少的工作。无论是初写者还是经验丰富的作者,在初稿完成后都要经过一番审读、推敲、修改才能定稿。实际上,完成初稿只是完成写作的一半工作。修改是对初稿内容的进一步深化和提高,对文字的进一步加工和润色,对观点的进一步订正。

修改论文可以从以下几个方面着手:

(1) 文题是否精炼、达意,内容是否切题。

(2) 论点是否鲜明,论据是否充分,论证是否严密。

(3) 框架结构是否合理,层次是否条理分明。

(4) 摘要是否反映全文的主旨。

(5) 数据是否准确。

(6) 结果是否支持结论,结论是否科学客观。

(7) 参考文献是否权威,是否有代表性和针对性。

(8) 量、单位及用词是否规范。

(9) 文稿是否符合医学论文写作规范或稿约要求。

(10) 标点符号是否正确,有无错别字,等等。

修改过程中,具体可以采取以下做法:

1. 通读全文,全局着眼　修改时,首先应该多看几遍文章,以便从整体上把握文章的内容和布局。局部的修改要从全局出发,要从整篇文章的具体语言环境中考虑如何修改字、词、句、段。文章的前后连贯、交代照应、过渡等修改,也必须纵观全局,立足全篇。

2. 查阅文献,澄清问题　对材料和结果要细心核对,对论点、论据、论证要提炼深化,使论点突出、论据充分。发现问题或可疑之处一定要查阅文献,核对清楚,主观臆断往往会出差错。

3. 虚心请教,忍痛割爱　自己写出来的东西,有时候即使感觉并不十分满意,也舍不得删改。但一个人的思维毕竟是有限的,而且往往带有主观色彩。初稿里的问题往往或因当局者迷,或因敝帚自珍,自己不容易发现,而旁观者清,常常能够看出其中的问题。所以,论文初稿完成后,最好请相关领域的专家评阅,并根据他们的意见进行修改。

4. 放声朗读,边读边改　一带而过地看文章,不容易发现句子是否通畅、用词是否准确、音调是否和谐等问题。放声朗读,口诵耳听,更容易发现较隐蔽的问题。

5. 反复修改,精益求精　一篇文章往往需要反复修改,逐字逐句推敲全文,大到内容结构,小到标点措辞,都应仔细审视,力求一错不漏。要有"百炼成字,千炼成句"的精神,反复修改,删去可有可无的语句,使得文字简练,语句平朴易懂。

（陈战）

第六节 论文投稿的流程和注意事项

一、期刊论文投稿流程

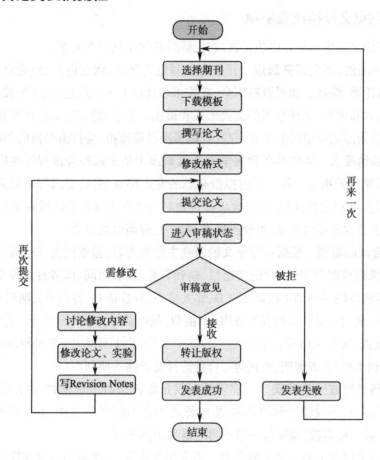

在投稿之前,作者首先要选择期刊,下载模板。需要注意的是,每个期刊都有自己的风格和特点,我们需要筛选出符合自己研究领域的期刊,这样写出来的论文更容易被期刊接受、发表。期刊成百上千,每个期刊都有自己的要求。通常来说,期刊的主页上都可以下载论文的写作模板和要求,我们可以根据模板和要求撰写论文。

论文初稿完成以后,可以根据论文模板和要求再次核对和修改论文格式,避免因格式不符合要求,而被期刊拒稿。

论文定稿以后,就要进行投稿了。大多数期刊都可以通过在线系统或电子邮箱提交论文。不同的期刊其审稿时间有所不同,有的需要一周,有的需要一个月,最长的一般不超过三个月,只需要静心等待即可。

审完稿后,期刊编辑会与作者取得联系。这时可能会出现三种情况。第一种情况是,论文质量较高,会被直接接受,然后签署转让版权协议,向杂志社支付版面费后,就可以等待论文发表了。这是最好的结果。第二种情况是，编辑会对稿件提出修改意见和要求，与作者讨论修改内容，这时只需要按照编辑的要求进行修改即可。修改之后，再次提交论文，等待审稿。一般论文不会一次性通过，需要进行多次修改。第三种情况是，论文水平达不到发表要求，投稿被拒，此次发表失败。作者可以考虑转投其他期刊，开始新一轮的投稿。

二、期刊论文投稿注意事项

要想提高论文写作水平并成功发表，在投稿时必须注意以下问题：

1. **要循序渐进，不要好高骛远** 开始时多写短篇报道、调查报告、经验介绍等，掌握一定技巧后再写论著、综述。如果资料不全，在技术和理论上无先进性，就不要硬写成论文，应根据掌握的资料和内容，选择适当的文稿形式和篇幅。初学撰稿者，稿件最好投寄级别较低的医学刊物，被录用的概率可能要高一些，否则多次投稿遭拒，会打击写稿的积极性。

2. **注意稿约要求** 稿约是各种医学杂志编辑部为使来稿符合该刊的性质、任务、内容的编排格式而制定的指导文件。了解拟投杂志的专业特点、稿约要求等非常重要。每种刊物选文均有侧重点和特色，即办刊宗旨。各刊物对稿件有不同的要求或在不同的时期需要不同的稿件，了解这些稿约要求，可使投稿有的放矢，提高登载机会。

3. **选择合适的期刊** 根据所写论文的研究主题和内容，检索同类或相似论文的发表情况，将检索结果列成期刊清单（含论文题目、期刊名称、发表时间、作者姓名及单位等），综合考虑期刊的类别（SCI 分区 /EI 检索、CSCD、北大核心、科技核心、普刊等）、期刊审稿 / 出版周期（初审、复审、录用到见刊等时长）、费用（审稿费、版面费等）、影响因子等。此外，还需了解期刊的栏目设置、文章风格等。结合论文的学术水平（创新性大小、理论深度等）和个人的发表需要（期刊水平、发表周期、费用等），合理选择要投稿的期刊。

4. **不一稿多投或一投多稿** 一稿多投不仅是版权法明令禁止的，也是各家刊物严防的。因为一稿多投，不仅浪费刊物资源，影响作者和刊物的声誉，也挫伤读者的感情。故而一旦发现有作者一稿多投，编辑部一般不再轻易采用其来稿。

另外，一投多稿也不利于论文的发表。不少作者认为，一次给同一家刊物投多篇论文可以提高命中率。其实不然。原因在于：第一，作者的多篇论文质量有差异，编辑部往往择其中质量较高的一篇进入审稿流程，其他的就可能放弃不用；第二，出于多种因素的考虑，编辑部一般不会连续刊发同一作者的论文；第三，多篇论文一起投，容易让编辑产生"多产而质量不高"的印象，最后非但不能"多投多中"，还很可能"多投少中"，甚至是"多投不中"。

5. **注意格式的规范** 不少报刊编辑部对稿件格式都有详细而明确的要求，投稿前要认真研究。一般而言，论文都有标题、通讯地址、邮政编码、作者姓名等。正文之前通常有200~300 字的摘要和3~5 个关键词。正文之后还应注明参考文献。有的还要求在文后加"作者简介"，以方便编辑了解情况，建立作者档案。

（陈战）

第二章　英文医学论文的结构与写作

第一节　文　题

一、文题的写作要求

文题(title)是论文的点睛之笔,是"一篇论文区别于其他论文的显著标记",影响着论文的第一印象和被检索度,因此撰写和翻译论文文题是一门艺术。好的文题应该具有准确、简洁、清楚的特点,用最精简的语言充分表述论文的主题和核心内容。

1. 准确(Accuracy)　作为论文的标签,文题应该尽可能涵盖论文的主要内容,确保含义准确,避免空泛;用词应该具有专指性,避免非定量的、含义不明的词(如 some、certain、rapid、new、novel 等)。

试比较以下文题:

① Action of antibiotics on bacteria

② Observations on the effect of certain antibiotics on various species of bacteria

③ Action of streptomycin on *Mycobacterium tuberculosis*

④ Inhibition of growth of *Mycobacterium tuberculosis* by streptomycin

从形式上看,文题①简短无冗词,但 antibiotics 和 bacteria 所指意义过于空泛;文题②中的 certain 和 various 不具有专指性,意义空泛;文题③列出了具体研究对象,准确性大为提高;文题④将文题③中的 Action of 具体化,含义更为准确。

2. 简洁(Brevity)　文题应该言简意赅,以最少的文字概括尽可能多的内容。文题一般不超过 10~12 个单词或 100 个英文字符(含空格和标点),长度尽量限制在一行之内,过长的文题会削弱读者对论文核心内容的印象。

文题中常可删去不必要的冠词(a,an 和 the)和多余的说明性词汇以实现简洁化,如 Research on、Analysis of、Development of、Evaluation of、Studies of/on、Experimental/Preliminary study、Observations on、Investigation of/on、Regarding、Report of/on、The preparation of 等。

试比较以下文题:

① The technique of nucleic acid test to detect HBV infection in blood donors

② Nucleic acid testing to detect HBV infection in blood donors

文题②用动名词 testing 替代文题①中的 The technique of...test,意思完全相同但形式更为简洁。

3. 清楚(Clarity)　文题应该清晰地反映文章的具体内容和特色,明确表明研究工作的独到之处,力求简洁有效、重点突出,因此应尽量将表达核心内容的主题词放在文题开头。例如:

Prospective natural-history study of coronary atherosclerosis,重点说明论文做的是前瞻性自然史研究(prospective natural-history study),而非其他类型的研究;

The effects of dietary and herbal phytochemicals on drug transporters,重点说明研究的对象是疗效(effect),而非 dietary and herbal phytochemicals 或者 drug transporters。

为实现文题的清晰性,应该慎重使用缩略语,除了某些国际公认的缩略语,如 DNA、RNA、mRNA 等在生物医学领域的文章中可直接使用外,一般期刊都规定缩略语首次出现时应使用全称,然后在圆括号内标注缩略语。例如:

Traditional Chinese medicine(TCM):are polyphenols and saponins the key ingredients triggering biological activities?

中医(TCM)是中国文化中的常见术语,但在英文期刊中首次出现时应该使用全称,然后在圆括号内标注缩略语。

二、英文文题的句式结构

英语医学论文的文题主要有 3 种句式结构,即词组式、陈述式和疑问式。

1. 词组式　词组式文题是英语医学论文文题中最常见的形式,这种形式简明醒目,易于突出主题。一般由一个名词或多个并列的名词,加上必要的修饰语构成,没有谓语成分,其中的动词多以分词或动名词形式出现。

例 1　Traditional Chinese medicine formulas for irritable bowel syndrome:from ancient wisdoms to scientific understandings

从古老智慧和现代科学看中药配方治疗肠易激综合征

例 2　Effects of Jianpi Qinghua formula on insulin resistance in type 2 diabetes mellitus rats by regulating transcription and inflammatory factors of intestinal tract Th1 and Th17

健脾清化方调节肠道 Th1 和 Th17 免疫细胞型转录因子及炎症因子改善 2 型糖尿病大鼠胰岛素抵抗

2. 陈述式　陈述式文题在英语医学期刊中偶尔出现,多用于陈述事实,或提出呼吁。常用结构为主谓式完整句,只是句尾没有句号。

例 3　Asymptomatic stage of human immunodeficiency virus infection is the optimal timing for its management with traditional Chinese medicine

人类免疫缺陷病毒感染的无症状阶段是中医药治疗的最佳时机

例 4　Coffee and herbal tea consumption is associated with liver stiffness in the general population:The Rotterdam study

普通人群中饮用咖啡和凉茶与肝硬度相关:一项鹿特丹研究

3. 疑问式　疑问式文题在英语医学期刊中偶尔出现,多用于评论性论文,其作用是使文题显得生动,以吸引读者。常用结构可以是句子也可以是词组,句尾要有问号(句子若以

when、what、where、who、how 等疑问代词或疑问副词开头,问号可以省略)。例如:

例 5　Should treatment for heart failure with preserved ejection fraction differ from that for heart failure with reduced ejection fraction?

要区别对待射血分数正常心力衰竭患者与射血分数降低心力衰竭患者吗?

例 6　Health related quality of life:is it another comprehensive evaluation indicator of Chinese medicine on acquired immune deficiency syndrome treatment?

健康相关生活质量是否是中医对获得性免疫缺陷综合征治疗的又一综合评价指标?

三、英文文题的书写格式

英文文题的书写格式主要有以下三种,但最终还要根据期刊的具体要求决定采用哪种格式。

1. 大写文题中所有实词的首字母　这是比较常见的书写格式,但要注意的是 5 个或 5 个以上字母的虚词亦要大写首字母。

例 7　Relationship Between Molecular Structure and Cytochrome P_{150} Metabolic Intermediate Complex Formation

2. 大写文题中第一个单词的首字母　此种格式自然、醒目,避免了虚词的大小写之争。

例 8　Patient blinding with blunt tip placebo acupuncture needles:comparison between 1mm and 2mm skin press

3. 大写文题中所有单词的所有字母　这是较为少见的书写方式,给人一种庄重、严肃的感觉。

例 9　HOW TO PREVENT RENAL TRAUMA

四、副文题的格式及作用

医学英语论文中常出现副文题,是对正文题的补充和说明。在文题内容层次较多、难以简化的情况下,主副文题格式具有层次清楚、逻辑简明的优点,被国际一流期刊广泛采用。正副文题的书写格式一般有三种:以冒号隔开、以圆点隔开、独立式。当今期刊最流行的格式是以冒号隔开,当文题只大写第一个单词的首字母时,副文题中的首字母可以大写也可小写。

副文题的作用是突出论文的一些主要内容,如病例数、研究方法、重点内容、同位关系、提出疑问等。

1. 突出病例数

例 10　Surgical treatment of pancreatic pseudocysts:analysis of 119 cases

119 例假性胰腺囊肿手术治疗

例 11　A multivariate analysis of long-term kidney graft survival:a clinical review of 2,016 cases

影响肾移植长期存活的多因素分析——2 016 例肾移植回顾

2. 突出研究方法

例 12　Review on the characteristics of liver-pacifying medicinal in relation to the treatment of stroke:from scientific evidence to traditional medical theory

从科学证据和传统医学理论角度回顾平肝药治疗中风的特点

例 13 Effect of conventional medical treatment plus Qigong exercise on type 2 diabetes mellitus in Chinese patients: a meta-analysis

常规治疗和气功对中国 2 型糖尿病患者疗效的荟萃分析

3. 突出重点内容

例 14 Sepsis: definition, epidemiology, and diagnosis

脓毒症的定义、流行病学和诊断

例 15 Drugs for the poor of the third world: consumption and distribution

向第三世界穷困人口提供药品的使用与分配

4. 表示同位关系

例 16 Alzheimer's disease: an emerging affliction of aging population

阿尔茨海默病是老年人群中新兴的疾病

例 17 Elevated intra-abdominal pressure in acute decompensated heart failure: a potential contributor to worsening renal function

急性失代偿性心力衰竭患者的腹内压升高是肾功能恶化的潜在因素

5. 提出疑问

例 18 Hyperglycemia in acute coronary syndromes: risk-marker or therapeutic target?

急性冠脉综合征中的高血糖: 风险标记还是治疗靶点?

例 19 Chronic abdominal pain: a surgical or psychiatric symptom?

慢性腹痛是手术症状还是精神症状?

五、英文文题的常用表达

(一) 常用词汇

1. 研究 a study/an analysis/a report/a research on+ 研究内容; a study/report of+ 案例数。

例 20 Genome-wide association study on susceptibility genes associated with yang-deficiency constitution

阳虚体质易感基因的全基因组关联研究

例 21 The recurrence and survival of oral squamous cell carcinoma: a report of 275 cases

275 例口腔鳞状细胞癌的复发存活率研究

例 22 Literature research on diagnosis-treatment rule for stroke of Danxi School

丹溪学派中风病诊治规律文献研究

2. 疗效 / 药效研究 effect/efficacy/impact of

例 23 Therapeutic effect of Guijiajiao (Colla Carapax et Plastrum Testudinis) on bone regeneration in rats and zebrafish

龟甲胶对大鼠和斑马鱼骨再生的治疗作用

例 24 TCM differentiation, treatment on IgA nephropathy and the efficacy evaluation

IgA 肾病中医辨证规律、治疗方法和疗效评价研究

例 25 Impact of Wentong Huoxue Cream on p-AKT protein expression in dorsal root ganglia in rats with diabetic peripheral neuropathy

温通活血乳膏对糖尿病周围神经病变大鼠背根神经节中 p-AKT 蛋白表达的影响

3. A 与 B 的关系 根据"简洁"的原则,"and"句式可代替 relationship。例如：

例 26 Malignant hypertension and cigarette smoking

恶性高血压与吸烟的关系

例 27 Glucose metabolism and coronary heart disease

糖代谢与冠心病的关系

(二)习惯用语

prospective study/survey/evaluation 前瞻性研究 / 调查 / 评价

retrospective study/survey/analysis 回顾性研究 / 调查 / 分析

a review of 综述

comparison/contrast between 比较

advances in the treatment of 治疗进展

a collaborative survey of 协作研究

an offspring study 子代研究

a history of progress 发展史

historical perspectives and future directions 历史回顾和展望

diagnostic and therapeutic technology assessment 诊断和治疗技术的评价

a meta-analysis 荟萃分析

a 30-week randomized double blind controlled trial 一项 30 周随机、双盲、对照试验

primary prevention trial and follow-up study 一级预防试验和随访研究

练习

1. 请将下列文题改为主副文题的格式。

(1) A light and electron microscopic study of 2 cases of primary sarcoma of the heart

(2) Experimental study of laser surgery of the liver

(3) Clinical analysis of 55 cases of subacute thyroiditis

(4) Evidence-based medicine is a new approach to teaching the practice of medicine

(5) Is autophagy in cell death an innocent convict?

2. 请将下列文题翻译成英语。

(1) 从三焦气化论肿瘤的中医病机

(2) 302 例慢性阻塞性肺疾病急性加重期中医证候分型

(3) CiteSpace 应用对 Web of Science 近 5 年针灸相关文献的计量学及可视化分析

> （4）传统运动疗法干预对膝骨关节炎患者疼痛改善及关节功能影响的系统评价
>
> （5）丹红注射液联合常规疗法治疗脑梗死患者的临床疗效及安全性 Meta 分析

（徐丽）

第二节 署名与单位

论文作者的署名权（authorship）目前并没有统一的定义，一般来讲，作者是指对某项研究做出突出贡献的个人或者为已发表的研究论文做出实质性学术研究贡献的人。国际医学期刊编辑委员会的署名权指导方针为"凡称为作者的个人均应符合作为作者的条件，凡符合资格的人士均应列出"。国际上对于作者资格有严格标准，如果研究者实际参与了以下工作，包括提出观点或设计实验、积极参与研究活动、分析和解释资料、撰写文章等，则均可以要求署名权。

而根据温哥华格式的定义，论文的作者则应同时满足以下三个条件：参与选题和设计，或参与资料的分析和解释者；起草或修改论文中关键性理论或其他主要内容者；能对编辑部意见进行核修，在学术上进行答辩，并最终同意论文发表者。以上三个条件缺一不可。

多数期刊对署名人数有限制，通常要求不超过 6 人，必要时也可稍加。对于不符合作者署名要求，但对论文做出一定的贡献者，可以在论文致谢（acknowledgement）中列出姓名及主要贡献，如资料收集、图表制作、数据统计等。

一、署名顺序

署名顺序是指根据对研究工作和论文撰写的贡献大小对论文作者进行的排序，一旦确定后不可随意改动或增减。通常情况下，除通讯作者外，贡献越大，排名越靠前。因此，多数论文对署名的顺序有严格规定，要求在投稿时写明每一位作者在本研究中的具体贡献。在英文论文中，应着重注意区分第一作者和通讯作者。

1. **第一作者（First Author）** 第一作者是科研课题的具体操作者和论文执笔者。一般是对研究工作做出最大贡献的人员，也是对论文的科学性和真实性承担主要责任者。

2. **通讯作者（Corresponding Author）** 通讯作者是指实际统筹处理投稿和承担答复审稿意见等工作的主导者。通常是科研团队和课题研究工作的主要负责人，除了课题的经费、实验设计、论文撰写和把关等工作之外，还要承担与编辑部的联系以及接受读者咨询等工作。因此，在英文期刊的要求中，通讯作者虽然一般位列于作者名单的最后，却是研究成果的主要拥有者，而第一作者只是研究的具体承担者、主要参与者和最大贡献者。在很多情况下，通讯作者和第一作者可能是同一个人。

二、署名格式

在对论文署名时，应注意格式的规范完整，主要包括作者姓名、学位和单位。

1. 作者姓名 英文期刊一般要求署名时使用全名,按照英语人名的顺序,名在前,姓在后,这一点应与参考文献的写法区分开来。

例如:Sabina White、Alfred Bernhard Nobel 等。当然,有些情况下,署名也会使用缩写,但是只是缩写名,不能缩写姓氏,缩写后要将名放在后面,且省略缩写点,或者也可将缩写后的名放在前,姓氏放在后面,此时应保留缩写点。

例如:

Caitriona Ryan 可以缩写为 Ryan C 或 C. Ryan。

James A. de Lemos 可以缩写为 de Lemos JA 或 J. A. de Lemos。

汉语姓名的署名格式基本遵循相似的规则,但通常不使用缩写点。如果姓名只有两个汉字,则将姓和名颠倒顺序并以拼音形式写出,且大写每个音节的首字母。例如:

刘斌,可以写作 Bin Liu。

如果姓名多于两个字,则只大写姓和名第一个字的首字母即可,名的两个字之间可以不空格或使用连字符连接。例如:

张广华,可以写作 Guanghua Zhang 或 Guang-hua Zhang。如果缩写的话,可以分别缩写为 Zhang G 和 Zhang GH。

可见,为避免文献检索时造成不必要的误解,后一种写法更值得推荐。具体采用哪种署名方式,建议作者参考拟投期刊的要求。另外,作者应尽量采用相对固定的英文署名,以增加在文献检索和论文引用中的准确性。

2. 作者学位 为避免姓名相同造成的文献识别混乱,有些医学期刊会要求在作者署名时标明学位。此时,使用缩写形式即可。常用的学位缩写如下:

M. B.(MB)=Bachelor of Medicine 医学学士

M. M.(MM)=Master of Medicine 医学硕士

M. S.(MS)=Master of Surgery 外科硕士

M. D.(MD)=Doctor of Medicine 医学博士

Ph. D.(PhD)=Doctor of Philosophy 博士 / 哲学博士

例如在 Alfred Bernhard Nobel,MD 中,Alfred Bernhard Nobel 是作者姓名,MD 则表明作者是医学博士。

3. 作者单位 根据作者排序,逐一列出各位作者的工作单位或就读学校、地址、邮政编码和国家,并使用上标符号标明与相应作者的关系。通讯作者还需列出详细地址、电话号码、电子邮箱等联系方式。常见通讯地址表达方式如下:

部门、科、处 division

科、系 department

研究所、学院 institute

部门、处、组 section

实验室 laboratory

病理学教研室 Department of Pathology

药学院 College of Pharmacy

防疫站 Anti-Epidemic Station

妇幼保健院 Maternal and Child Health Care Institute

附属医院 Affiliated Hospital

省第三人民医院 Provincial NO. 3 People's Hospital

省卫生厅 Provincial Health Bureau

县医院 County Hospital

中医医院 Hospital of Traditional Chinese Medicine

胸科医院 Chest Hospital

教学医院 Teaching Hospital

综合医院 General Hospital

针灸研究所 Institute of Acupuncture and Moxibustion

中国红十字总会 Red Cross Society of China

中华医学会 Chinese Medical Association

例如：

Division of Newborn Medicine, Department of Pediatrics, the Mount Sinai School of Medicine, New York, NY, USA.（美国西奈山医学院儿科学系新生儿科）

　　注意，如果论文作者为两位或两位以上，署名时需要使用逗号将每位作者姓名隔开，并在最后一位作者姓名前使用 and；如果出现其中两位作者贡献相同，无法区分排名，或者第一作者同时也是通讯作者等情况，也可以使用"*"等上标符号予以说明。

三、论文署名示例

Vascular Endothelial Growth Factor Overexpression Prolongs Survival in Amyotrophic Lateral Sclerosis Mice

Hong Tang[1*], Xiao Wang[2], Jian Shen[3] and Surita Banwait[4]

1. Department of Neurology, University of California, SF, CA 94121, USA

2. Department of Neurology and Institute of Neurology, Ruijin Hospital, Shanghai Jiao Tong University School of Medicine, Shanghai 200040, China

3. Department of Neurosurgery, Huashan Hospital, Fudan University, Shanghai 200040, China

4. Department of Neurosurgery, First Affiliated Hospital, Zhejiang Medical University, Zhejiang 100030, China

*Correspondence to Hong Tang MD, PhD

Tel：415-555-8769

Fax：425-555-8769

Email：Hongtang@ucsf.edu

学术论文的署名不仅是一种荣誉，更是一种责任。署名的同时即相当于发出一项声明，署名中的作者对论文拥有著作权，任何单位和个人不得侵犯。同时，署名也意味着文责自负，对论文的科学性和真实性负有不可推卸的责任。因此，署名问题看似简单，实则不然，为避免日后出现争议和纠纷，应仔细斟酌而定，不可随意为之。

练习 ✒

假设你和你的团队正在进行一项题为 Psychosocial Working Conditions and the Utilization of Health Care Services 的研究，请写出以此题目所撰写论文的署名，研究团队人员姓名、地址等信息可自拟。

（曲悝　徐丽）

第三节　摘　要

一、摘要的定义和作用

国内外学界对论文摘要的定义：

An abstract is defined as an abbreviated, accurate representation of the content of a document, preferably prepared by its author(s) for the publication with it. Such abstracts are also useful in access publications and machine-readable data bases.

（The American National Standards Institute, 1979）

An abstract should be viewed as a mini-version of the paper. An abstract should provide a brief summary of each of the main sections of the paper: Introduction, Materials and Methods, Results and Discussion. As Houghton (1975) puts it, "An abstract can be defined as a summary of the information in a document."

（Day, 1998）

An abstract is a complete but concise and informative account of your work, i. e. a condensation that makes sense without reference to the full document. It is not merely a descriptive guide to the content of the paper, but rather it is an abbreviated version of the paper (except for very long review-style papers or monographs, in which descriptive abstracts may be used.)

（Tippett, 2004）

摘要是对报告、论文的内容不加注释和评论的简短陈述。报告、论文一般应有摘要,为了国际交流,还应有外文(多用英文)摘要。

(GB7713-87)

国外学界分别用"代表"(representation)、"概括"(summary)和"报告"(account)三个词汇描述摘要的定义,其本质意思和 GB7713-87 的规定是一致的,即摘要是对研究论文的简要陈述和概括,是论文内容的浓缩与精华。

摘要展示了论文的研究主题和框架,是论文的关键部分之一。联合国教科文组织明确规定:"全世界公开发表的论文,无论用何种文字写成,必须随附一篇简短的英文摘要。"当今数字出版时代,摘要是读者最先得到并且可能是唯一能够免费获得的信息。一篇好的摘要能够让读者快速、准确地检索到论文的主要内容,不仅决定着读者是否需要进行全文阅读,也直接影响着论文的被引用情况。

二、摘要的类型

由于研究内容与方法上的差异,论文摘要大致可以分为信息性摘要(informative abstract)和描述性摘要(descriptive abstract)。

1. 信息性摘要 也被称为报道性摘要或资料性摘要,通常是一篇完整的短文,相当于论文的简介或概要,阐明研究问题和主要研究成果,但它又不是对原文篇幅简单的缩减,需要进行深入加工。信息性摘要全面、简要地概括论文的目的、方法、主要数据和结论,充分反映论文的创新之处。这类摘要语言精炼、内容简明、信息量大,是一篇正文的微缩版。阅读摘要可以部分取代阅读全文。

目前大部分科技期刊和会议论文都要求作者提供结构式摘要,这实质上是报道性摘要的结构化。一般包括:背景(context/background)、目的(objective)、设计(design)、地点(setting)、对象(participants/patients/subjects/samples)、处理方法(interventions)、主要结果测定指标(main outcome measures)、结果(results)和结论(conclusion)等。目前国内外医学期刊中,结构式摘要较统一的项目包括:目的(objective/aim)、背景(background)、方法(methods)、结果(results)及结论(conclusion),具体格式请参照期刊要求。例如:

Abstract:Background Neonatal jaundice affects at least 481,000 newborns every year. Phototherapy is recommended but its effects are limited and adverse reactions can occur. In China,…Yinzhihuang oral liquid and phototherapy was compared to phototherapy alone for treating neonatal jaundice. **Methods** A comprehensive literature search was performed in four Chinese databases,two English language databases and two trial registries from inception to June 2017.…Data were analyzed using RevMan 5.3. **Results** Totally 17 trials(involving 2,561 neonates) were included in this review. 14 of them had a high risk of bias. Significant differences were detected between combination therapy and phototherapy alone for serum bilirubin level(MD −50.25μmol/L, 95% CI −64.01 to −36.50,I^2=98%;7 trials,post-hoc decision choosing random effects model)…reached the required information size(DARIS=1,301 participants). **Conclusion** Based on trials with low methodological quality, Yinzhihuang oral liquid combined with phototherapy seemed to be safe and superior to phototherapy alone for reducing serum bilirubin in neonatal jaundice. These potential benefits need to be confirmed in future trials using rigorous methodology.

2. 描述性摘要 也被称为指示性摘要(indicative abstract)或论点摘要(topic abstract),只描述论文或报告的主题思想,不涉及或很少涉及细节问题,但要指示文献的主题和所取得成果的性质和水平,使读者对该研究内容有大概的了解,决定是否需要进一步查阅原文。

描述性摘要的优点是文字简短、言简意赅,通常只用四五句话概括论文或报道的主题,常用于综述性论文、会议报告和艺术评论等;其突出的缺点是信息量较少,一般实验性论文很少使用指示性摘要。例如:

Abstract: Although lots of great achievements have been gained in the battle against cancer during the past decades, cancer is still the leading cause of death in the world including developing countries such as China. Traditional Chinese medicine (TCM) is popular in Chinese and East Asian societies as well as some other Western countries and plays an active role in the modern healthcare system including patients with cancer, which may act as a potential effective strategy in treating human cancers. In this review, we aimed to introduce the mechanisms of TCM compound, as an option of individualized therapy, in treating cancer patients from the perspective of both Chinese and Western medicine. Therefore, TCM compound plays a critical role in treating patients with cancer, which has a promising strategy in the field of cancer management.

三、英文摘要的写法

(一)目的(Objective/Aim)

论文摘要中的"目的"部分应该用一两句话概括研究工作的前提、目的及主题范围,须具有高度的简明性、完整性、科学性、检索性和准确性。描述性英文摘要一般用完整的句子保持语篇照应,结构式摘要则多用动词不定式短语,完整句子相对较少。

1. 完整句子常用表达

- The purpose/aim of the study/review/this paper/investigation is/was to...

- The objectives of this study were to.../The present study is an attempt to...

- A retrospective investigation was designed/undertaken to...

时态:介绍一般性资料、现象或普遍事实时,多使用一般现在时;使用 however、but、yet、few、little、no 等指出过去研究的不足并引出作者的研究问题时,使用现在完成时;叙述本人或他人近期的工作时,采用过去时。

例 1 The purpose of this study was to examine the association between acute plaque rupture and exertion-related sudden coronary death in a series of carefully studied autopsy hearts.

本研究的目的是通过详细的心脏解剖检查,研究急性斑块破裂与用力导致的冠状动脉性猝死之间的联系。

例 2 This retrospective study was designed to evaluate clinico-pathological data including results of treatment and prognostic factors which affect the overall survival and disease-free survival.

　　该回顾性研究旨在评估影响总体生存率和无病生存率的临床病理资料,包括治疗效果和预后因素。

　　2. 不定式常用表达　注意:Aim/Objective 可以大写首字母或大写全部字母,其后可接冒号或省略冒号。具体格式请参照期刊要求。

　　● 探讨:To discuss/find/observe/investigate/explore/probe...

　　例 3　**AIM** To investigate the changes of the contents of lead and selenium in the whole blood, feces and urine of rats with lead poisoning.

探讨铅中毒对大鼠全血、粪便与尿液中微量元素铅和硒的变化。

　　例 4　**Objective** To observe the effect and safety of Hongjingtian (Rhodiola) capsule in treating mild or moderate major depressive disorder with deficiency of both heart and spleen.

观察红景天胶囊治疗轻中度抑郁症心脾两虚证的疗效及安全性。

　　● 报告:To report the result/experience of...

　　例 5　**AIM** To report the authors' experience in performing adult-to-adult living donor liver transplantation (LDLT) by using a modified technique in the grafts of the right lobe of the liver.

报告使用肝脏右叶移植新技术进行成人间活体肝移植的经验。

　　● 评估:To evaluate/assess the effect/relationship/mechanism of...

　　例 6　**OBJECTIVE** To evaluate the clinical efficacy of Liuwei Dihuang capsule in the treatment of liver-kidney yin deficiency syndrome in N of 1, randomized controlled, double blind trial.

单病例随机对照双盲试验评价六味地黄胶囊治疗肝肾阴虚证的临床疗效。

　　例 7　**AIM** To assess the likelihood ratios of diagnostic strategies for pulmonary embolism and to determine their clinical application according to pretest probability.

评估肺栓塞诊断策略的似然比,并通过验前概率评价其临床应用价值。

　　● 阐明:To reveal/clarify/elucidate...

　　例 8　**Aim**: To elucidate the efficacies of tolvaptan (TLV) as a treatment for refractory ascites compared with conventional treatment.

与传统治疗方法相比较,阐明使用托伐普坦治疗顽固性腹水的效力。

　　● 比较:To compare...with...

　　例 9　**Objective** To compare the image quality, dose, diagnostic value of perspective ECG-triggering with retrospective ECG gating coronary artery computed tomography.

比较前瞻性心电门控与回顾性心电门控冠状动脉 CT 的图像质量、辐射剂量及诊断价值。

　　● 回顾:To review/summarize/study/analyze/retrospectively...

　　例 10　**Aim** To review the current knowledge of persistent visual loss after non-ocular surgeries under general anesthesia.

回顾性分析当前关于全麻下非眼科手术后持续性视力丧失的现状。

例 11 **Objective** To retrospectively explore the diagnosis and treatment of postoperative lumbar intervertebral disc infection.

回顾性探讨腰椎间盘术后椎间隙感染的诊断与治疗方法。

● 建立：To establish/develop/construct a model/system/technique...

例 12 **Aim** To establish animal model of heart-qi deficiency syndrome by the method of comparative medicine.

用比较医学的方法建立心气虚证动物模型。

例 13 **Objective** To construct an eukaryotic expression plasmid containing gene coding of newcastle disease virus（NDV）oncolytic strain Italien.

构建天然溶瘤型新城疫病毒基因的真核表达载体。

例 14 **AIM**：To establish and compare the methods for culturing neonatal rat cardiac fibroblasts culture.

建立并比较新生大鼠心肌成纤维细胞的培养方法。

● 查明：To research/discover/ascertain...problem/evidence/material... 例如：

例 15 **Objective**：To research the problems about venous transfusion in out-patient clinic so as to improve the quality of nursing.

研究门诊静脉输液存在的问题，以提高护理质量。

例 16 **AIM**：To ascertain the acquisition of cytomegalovirus infection following exchange transfusion and factors affecting such transmission in newborn infants at a tertiary care hospital in India.

查明在印度第三级医疗机构中新生儿换血后巨细胞病毒感染以及影响感染的因素。

● 总结：To summarize/sum up...experience of...

例 17 **Objective**：To summarize diagnostic and therapeutic experience by analyzing the clinical features of serious type of acute virus myocarditis（SAVM）.

通过分析急性重症病毒性心肌炎的临床特点，总结诊治经验。

练习 1

请将下列句子翻译成英语。

（1）分析不同产地新鲜丹参中主要活性成分含量，合理评价鲜丹参药材品质。

（2）研究清热化湿祛瘀中药清肾颗粒治疗慢性肾衰竭湿热证患者的临床疗效。

（3）采用单病例随机对照双盲试验评价六味地黄胶囊治疗肝肾阴虚证的临床疗效，并评估该方法在证候疗效评价中的可应用性及可靠性。

（二）方法（Methods）

研究方法是实验研究或临床试验的手段，一般包括研究设计、研究对象、处理和测定方法、统计分析四个方面。英文写作时常用一般过去时表示回顾性叙述，且多用被动语态。

常用短语和句型

● 研究对象选择：were enrolled/selected

例18 111 patients with cerebral infarction who were admitted in 2003 were enrolled in this study.

研究收集了 2003 年全年收治入院的 111 例脑梗死患者的病历。

例19 60 patients with PGS after resection of esophageal cardiac cancer, admitted to the Second Affiliated Hospital of Nanjing Medical University from August 2012 to August 2015, were selected and studied randomly.

随机收集 2012 年 8 月至 2015 年 8 月南京医科大学第二附属医院的 60 名食管贲门癌切除术后 PGS 患者作为研究对象。

● 研究对象分组：were randomized into; were randomly divided/allocated/categorized into...

例20 60 patients were randomized into four groups: acupuncture-movement (AM) group, sham acupuncture-movement (SAM) group, conventional acupuncture (CA) group, and physical therapy (PT) group.

60 名患者随机分成四组：针刺运动（AM）组，假针刺运动（SAM）组，常规针刺（CA）组和物理治疗（PT）组。

例21 Totally 58 patients with ischemic post-stroke depression were randomly divided into two groups. The acupuncture group was given Tiaoshen Kaiqiao acupuncture therapy and placebo starch tablets treatment while the control group was treated with....

58 名缺血性脑卒中后抑郁患者随机分为两组。针灸组接受调肾开窍针灸疗法和淀粉安慰剂疗法，对照组……

例22 A total of 340 inpatients, aged 40–79 years, with exacerbating CHF from 10 hospitals were enrolled and randomly allocated within 24h of admission.

来自 10 家医院的 340 名心力衰竭加重的住院患者，年龄处于 40~79 岁，在入院后 24 小时内随机分组。

● （回顾性）分析：(retrospectively) analyze

例23 Methods: We retrospectively analyzed the clinical data of 150 patients with HCC from January 2005 to March 2009.

本研究回顾分析了 2005 年 1 月至 2009 年 3 月 150 名肝细胞癌患者的临床数据。

例24 Clinical data of patients with peripheral vascular complications were analyzed retrospectively.

对发生外周血管并发症患者的相关临床资料进行回顾性分析。

● 用……方法分离：was isolated by

例25 Neonatal rat hearts were isolated by collagenase+trypsin or trypsin digestion. The cardiomyocytes and cardiac fibroblasts were isolated by different attachment techniques.

分别通过胶原酶＋胰蛋白酶法和胰蛋白酶消化法对新生大鼠心肌组织进行分离，利用贴壁时间差分离心肌细胞和心肌成纤维细胞。

- 用……方法测定、测量：was measured/detected/determined by

例 26 Patients with CS(cervical spondylosis)were treated with acupuncture and measured with a pulse acquisition device based on image(PADBI)before the first and after the tenth acupuncture sessions.

颈椎病患者接受针灸治疗，并在第一次治疗之前和第十次治疗之后用基于图像的脉冲采集装置（PADBI）进行测量。

例 27 Patterns of tea drinking and temperature at which tea was drunk were measured among healthy participants in a cohort study.

在一项队列研究中测量健康受试者的饮茶模式及其饮用时的茶温。

- 诊断：was diagnosed through/on the basis of

例 28 11 cases were diagnosed through the operation examination, and 7 cases were diagnosed via the needle biopsy of pleura.

11 例外科手术活检确诊，7 例胸腔穿刺后确诊。

- 治疗：was treated with

例 29 21 cases were treated with decompression and anterior subcutaneous transposition of ulnar nerve, and other 26 cases were treated with decompression and anterior submuscular transposition of ulnar nerve.

21 例患者接受减压治疗和尺神经皮下前置术，另外 26 例接受减压治疗和尺神经肌下前置术。

练习 2

请将下列句子翻译成英语。

（1）将符合方案的 282 例患者分为试验组 136 例，对照组 146 例；试验组与对照组均采用基础治疗，试验组加用清肾颗粒，疗程为 12 周。

（2）最后，我们根据患者体重与疗效之间的关系分析了适合该疗法的患者群体。

（3）采用 LTQ-Orbitrap XL 高分辨质谱仪测定全国 7 个不同产地新鲜丹参中 5 个丹酚酸类和 12 个丹参酮类成分。

（三）结果（Results）

"结果"是对实验结果的详细描述，通常用实验数据说明实验前后的变化，相对篇幅较长，是摘要部分的核心。英文写作时应注意："结果"亦是回顾性陈述，除描述性说明外，一般用过去时态。

常用短语和句型

- 结果表明：The results/findings showed/suggested/indicated/demonstrated/revealed/documented that...;It was found to/that...;We found that...

例 30 Comparison between the acupuncture group and the Western medicine group for the curative rate on PSD(post-stroke depression)revealed an *OR* of 1.48,95% CI=[1.11 1.97]and *P*=0.008.

针灸组和西药组对 PSD(卒中后抑郁)治愈率的比较显示 *OR* 为 1.48,95%CI=[1.11 1.97],*P*=0.008。

例 31 This result indicated that the speed of symptom improvement decreased significantly after several acupuncture courses.

结果表明,几个针灸疗程之后症状改善的速度明显下降。

● 与……相比较:compared with

例 32 Compared with before the treatment,the scores on menstrual color and quantity, soreness and weakness of waist and knee,and breast swelling pain were decreased in both groups after treatment(*P*<0.05).

与治疗前比较,治疗后两组患者在月经颜色和数量、腰膝酸痛、乳房胀痛等方面评分均有所降低(*P*<0.05)。

例 33 Compared with the healthy group,the value of h5 was decreased significantly in the sub-healthy group(*P*<0.01).

与健康组比较,亚健康组的 h5 值显著降低(*P*<0.01)。

● 与……有关:was significantly/obviously associated/correlated with

例 34 Log-rank analysis identified expression of both CD90 and EpCAM was significantly associated with survival time of HCC patients.

CD90 和 EpCAM 的 Log-rank 分析鉴定表达与 HCC 患者的存活时间显著相关。

● 与……成正/反比:was directly/inversely proportional to

例 35 Results:fetal head was proportional to vertebral column under normal condition;CSD correlates well with BPD(*r*=0.982 7,*P*<0.001).The regression formula was CSD=6.45+1.53 BPD.

结果:在正常情况下,胎头和脊柱是相称的,CSD 与 BPD 之间有非常显著的正相关(*r*=0.982 7,*P*<0.001),回归方程为 CSD=6.45+1.53BPD。

● 增加与减少:was obviously/significantly increased/decreased in

例 36 After treatment,the VAS and RMDQ scores were significantly decreased in the three groups compared with before the treatment(*P*<0.05),and the improvements on scores in the combination group were better than those in the tendon group and the training group(*P*<0.05).

治疗后,三组患者 VAS 和 RMDQ 评分均较治疗前显著下降(*P*<0.05),联合治疗组评分提高幅度优于肌腱组和训练组(*P*<0.05)。

例 37 After treatment,the ACT score was obviously increased in both groups(*P*<0.05),and the IgE level was obviously decreased(*P*<0.05)and the frequency of asthma attack within one year was obviously reduced(*P*<0.05).

治疗后,两组 ACT 评分明显增加(*P*<0.05),IgE 水平明显降低(*P*<0.05),1 年内的哮喘发

作次数明显减少（*P*<0.05）。

● 有统计学意义、有显著差异：There was significant/statistical difference between...and...；Significant difference was found...

例 38 There was significant difference between the SERS（Side Effects Rating Scale）scores of two groups（*P*<0.05）；the control group had more adverse reactions，and the score would be increased with the extension of treatment time.

两组 SERS（副作用评定量表）评分差异有统计学意义（*P*<0.05）；对照组不良反应较多，随着治疗时间的延长，SERS 评分增加。

例 39 No significant difference was found in the time to alleviation of symptoms，incidence of complications，time to becoming afebrile，or rate of severe illness among the conventional groups and combination treatment groups.

在常规和联合治疗组中，症状缓解、并发症发生率、发热时间、重疾发生率之间没有显著差异。

练习 3

请将下列句子翻译成英语。

（1）同一产地新鲜丹参主要活性成分的含量基本一致，不同产地新鲜丹参主要活性成分的含量差异显著。

（2）试验组临床疾病总有效率为 79.41%，优于对照组 67.12%（*P*<0.05）。

（3）两组治疗 12 周后，对尿红细胞和各种指标的疗效无统计学差异。

（四）结论（Conclusion）

"结论"是作者对研究结果的综合分析，通常比较简短，用一两句话概括研究结果、局限性和未来展望。英文写作时应注意：如果结论具有普遍性，用一般现在时；如果结论为研究结束时的结论，不具备普遍性，则用一般过去式。

例 40 Jianpi Huayu decoction shows good clinical efficacy in the treatment of senile macular degeneration，which can enhance the antioxidant activity.

健脾化瘀汤治疗老年性黄斑变性临床疗效良好，可增强抗氧化能力。

例 41 In this large study，a modest increase in protein content and a modest reduction in the glycemic index led to an improvement in maintenance of weight loss.

在这项大规模研究中，适度增加蛋白含量和适度降低血糖指数能够促进体重减轻。

常用短语和句型

● 数据/结果说明/证实：The data/results suggested/showed/confirmed/demonstrated/indicated/revealed that...

例 42 The results suggested that Aidi injection could significantly improve the clinical effect of TAC and reduce the incidence of adverse events.

结果表明艾迪注射液可明显改善 TAC 的临床疗效,降低不良事件的发生率。

例 43　The result showed that the steady rate following the standard for evaluation of Karnofsky was over 87.0% in group B, 72.0% in Group A and 57.0% in Group C, respectively.

结果表明,遵循 Karnofsky 评价标准的稳定率在 B 组中超过 87.0%,在 A 组中为 72.0%,在 C 组中为 57.0%。

- 显著优于:be significantly better than

例 44　There was statistically significant difference on the clinical efficacy between the two groups, and the clinical efficacy of the treatment group was significantly better than that of the control group(P<0.05).

组间临床疗效比较,差异有统计学意义,治疗组显著优于对照组(P<0.05)。

- 描述疗效:shows good efficacy;can+ 动词原形

例 45　Bushen Shugan Huoxue recipe shows good clinical efficacy on hypomenorrhea following artificial abortion. It can obviously increase the menstrual volume and endometrium thickness of patients.

补肾疏肝活血方治疗人工流产术后月经过少的临床疗效良好,可明显增加患者的月经量和子宫内膜厚度。

例 46　Modified kinesio taping of integrated Chinese and Western medicine shows good efficacy in the treatment of knee osteoarthritis, which can obviously improve the active range of motion in knee joint of patients, and relieve the symptoms such as pain and stiffness.

中西医结合改良肌内效贴布治疗膝骨性关节炎的疗效满意,可明显改善患者膝关节自主活动度,减轻其疼痛、僵硬等症状。

- 本研究的重要贡献:A major new finding of this study is;Our findings elucidated/explored/explained...

例 47　In summary, our findings elucidated the potential mechanism of Baoyuan decoction on cardio-protection, and further explained its traditional efficacy in the molecular level.

综上所述,该研究阐释了保元汤发挥心肌保护作用的潜在药理机制,进而从分子细胞水平解释了保元汤的传统功效。

- 有必要做进一步的分析:Further analysis/trials are still needed to...;the results need to be further validated

例 48　However, there was potential bias in the included studies, so the conclusion still needed further high quality randomized controlled trials to improve the evidence level.

然而,本研究存在潜在偏倚,因此仍需要进行高质量的随机对照试验,以获取更多证据。

例 49　However, due to the lack of large-scale multi-center research, the results still need to be further validated in the clinic application.

但由于缺少大规模多中心研究,该结果还有待临床进一步验证。

● 建议、展望:should/may+ 动词原形

例 50 The overall quality of headache guidelines was low in China, but evidence-based guidelines are gradually becoming mainstream. Guideline developers should carefully consider, in particular, three domains:rigor of development, applicability, and editorial independence.

中国头痛指南的总体质量较低,但循证指南逐渐成为主流。指南制定者应特别仔细考虑以下三个领域:严格开发、适用性和独立编辑。

例 51 This novel method may provide a methodological reference for exploring the pharmacological mechanism of traditional Chinese formula in the future.

这种新方法可以为未来探索传统中药药理机制提供方法论参考。

练习 4

请将下列句子翻译成英语。

(1)结果表明中药治疗早期糖尿病肾病是安全有效的。

(2)单病例随机对照试验可应用于证候类中药的疗效评价,具有应用性及可靠性。

(3)清肾颗粒联合西医基础治疗对慢性肾衰竭湿热证患者在改善症状、降低证候积分值、减少尿蛋白、保护肾功能方面,显示了良好的临床疗效。

(徐丽)

第四节 关 键 词

关键词(keywords)是指论文文题、摘要和正文中重要的或反复出现的关键性单词或词组。关键词是文献搜索的重要依据,必须能够表达论文的中心内容。通常可以提取论文文题或摘要中的重点内容作为关键词,一般为 3~5 个词语或短语。

例 1 Title:Effects of Chinese herbs in children with Henoch-Schonlein purpura nephritis:a randomized controlled trial

Keywords:purpura;Schoenlein-Henoch;nephritis;Chinese herbs;randomized controlled trial

其中,关键词 purpura,Schoenlein-Henoch,nephritis,randomized controlled trial 提取于论文文题,关键词 Chinese herbs 提取于论文摘要。

例 2 Title:Efficacy and safety of Xinglou Chengqi decoction for acute ischemic stroke with constipation:study protocol for a randomized controlled trial

Keywords:Stroke;Constipation;Randomized controlled trial;Clinical protocols;Xinglou Chengqi decoction

其中,关键词 Stroke,Constipation,Randomized controlled trial,Xinglou Chengqi decoction 提取于论文文题,关键词 Clinical protocols 提取于论文摘要。

英语论文的关键词格式应注意以下几点：

（1）格式。具体格式请参照期刊规定，例如：Keywords:/KEY WORDS:/[Key words]

（2）词性。一般为名词或名词性词组，词语之间用逗号或者分号隔开，最后一个单词后面不加符号。

（3）大小写。除专有名词外，通常使用小写或只大写单词首字母。

（4）单复数。除特殊用法，英文名词一般用单数。

（5）正斜体。除拉丁学名或包含变量的词，一般用正体。

例如：

Keywords: epigallocate-echin-3-gallate; prostate cancer; survivin; proliferation

KEY WORDS: hepatocellular carcinoma; liver transplantation; living donor

[Key words]ECG-gating; Prospective; Retrospective; Congenital heart disease; CT

（徐丽）

第五节 引 言

引言（introduction）是论文正文的第一部分，篇幅相对较短，主要包括但不局限于以下内容：①研究背景和研究对象；②已有的研究成果及简单评价；③研究方法；④研究结果；⑤研究结论。

就英文写作而言，尤其要注意时态的使用。简言之，叙述研究对象的背景时，多使用一般现在时；叙述已有的研究成果时，多使用一般现在时和现在完成时；叙述本研究的内容和方法时，多使用一般过去时。与以往多使用被动语态不同的是，当前医学论文中亦会出现主动语态，使用 This study investigated/We investigated in this study... 等表达，明确动作的施动者，以积极的态度看待作者所从事的研究。

例 1 Chronic obstructive pulmonary disease (COPD) is a respiratory condition that manifests as central airway mucus hypersecretion, and peripheral airway reconstruction and scar tissue formation. The pathogenesis of COPD **is** complex, but the JAK/STAT signaling pathway and protease/anti-protease systems **play** an important role. COPD is also associated with matrix metalloproteinases (MMPs), and tissue inhibitor of metalloproteinase (TIMPs)（一般现在时，说明研究背景）. **Studies have shown that** the Janus kinase (JAK)/signal transducer and activator of transcription (STAT) signaling pathway can lead to the accumulation of a large number of proinflammatory cytokines, and increase the inflammatory response. The direct result of airway injury **is** lung tissue damage, which causes coughing, wheezing, and reduced lung function. MMP and TIMP expression imbalance causes degradation of extracellular matrix deposition disorder, which results in airway damage and emphysema （现在完成时和一般现在时，说明已有的研究结果）. This study **investigated** the expression and relationship between the JAK/STAT signaling pathway and MMPs/TIMPs in a rat model of COPD（一

般过去时,说明本研究的内容). Preclinical findings show that Liuwei Buqi capsules can not only reduce airway inflammation in patients with COPD, but also significantly improve cough, wheezing, shortness of breath, fatigue, and lung function in patients with COPD. In this study, a rat COPD model **was established** by administration of lipopolysaccharide and smoke. Liuwei Buqi capsules **were administered** after model establishment and lung function and lung tissue morphological changes, and changes in the STAT pathway and MMP system were observed (一般过去时,说明本研究的方法).

例2 Henoch-Schonlein purpura (HSP) **is** a systemic disease characterized by leukocytic vasculitis of small vessels and sediment of immunoglobulin A (IgA). Whether the kidney is affected is crucial for the prognosis of HSP in adolescent patients. When there is renal impairment, it is called Henoch-Schonlein purpura nephropathy (HSPN), which **accounts for** 78.9% of secondary glomerulopathy in children. The disease has a long illness course and can easily relapse into life-threatening late nephropathy in severe cases (一般现在时,说明研究对象背景). According to our earlier research, we **found** that the recipe prescribed by Professor Xueyi Pei (Traditional Chinese Medicine Department, Beijing Children's Hospital affiliated to Capital Medical University) for promoting diuresis, removing toxins, nourishing the kidney, and consolidating essence has a curative effect and is safe for HSPN in children (一般过去时,说明已有的研究结果). Therefore, we **carried out** a randomized controlled trial with a large sample size to study the curative effect of the recipe on HSPN. We also **aimed to** explore the pathological features of and curative effect on internal accumulation of damp-toxin, and seek the indications and mechanism of the therapy (一般过去时,说明本研究的方法与目的). This study **could** provide fewer toxic side-effects, standardize treatment, enhance curative effect, and improve prognosis over standard therapy in HSPN treatment (could 表示可能性,说明本研究的意义).

(徐丽)

第六节 材料与方法

一、综述

材料与方法(materials and methods)是论文正文的第二部分,是论文科学性的基础,是提供科学性研究的依据,旨在说明解决研究问题的技术路径,一方面为其他研究者提供参考和借鉴,另一方面也为研究成果的可靠性与可信性提供依据。因此,论文作者必须对研究的材料和方法进行全面而详尽的介绍,描述的详细程度应当以别人能够重复和再现文中的实验条件和结果为标准。

从写作的内容来看,材料部分要阐明研究过程中使用了什么;方法部分要阐明研究过程中做了什么,怎样做的以及为什么要这么做。

为了较为详尽地回答这些问题,目前越来越多的学术杂志要求论文中包含 Materials and

Methods,而不是单纯的 Methods。论文中所表述的"材料"应主要包括材料来源、性质、数量、选取及处理等。"方法"应当包括实验的仪器、设备、装置、实验条件、测试方法、分组情况、数理统计、误差分析等。其具体要求如下:

1. 对材料的描述应当清楚、准确 材料中应当清楚地指出研究对象(样品或者产品、动物、植物、患者)的数量、来源和准备方法。对于实验材料的名称,应当采用国际同行所熟悉的通用名称,尽量避免使用只有作者所在国家的人所熟悉的专门名称。

2. 对于方法的描述要详略得当、重点突出 应遵循的原则是提供足够的细节信息以便同行能够重复试验。避免混入有关结果或发现方面的内容。如果使用的方法属前人所用且众所周知或者业内人士公用的,只需提供方法名称;如属新的技术革新、实验设计、临床观察、手术等方法和手段,且未公开发表过,均需要详细阐述,并提供必要的细节;经过改进的,则重点写出改进部分和原方法的比较。

3. 引用他人的方法要注意文献出处 对已公开发表但尚未为人们所熟悉的方法,要提供文献出处,并对其方法原理作简单描述。

4. 统计等处理方法 应当介绍具体的统计方法,并包括统计学评价强度。

二、写作内容

1. 研究对象(Subject) 生物医学科技论文要求详细说明实验对象,包括正常人、患者、实验动物、组织、细胞等。以下分别加以说明,并介绍一些英语实例。

(1) 人体:包括人数、性别、年龄、健康状况、疾病状况等。临床研究的对象是患者,在使用患者的各种资料时,需有患者的同意,并通过伦理委员会批准。临床上,除上述基本情况外,还应说明来自住院部或门诊部,同时必须将病例数、职业、病因、病程、病理诊断依据、疾病诊断分型标准、分组标准、病情和治疗判断依据、观察方法和指标等情况作一一说明。除此以外,不同研究内容的论文还有不同的具体要求:①研究诊断方法的论文:要注意写明受试对象是否包括了各类不同患者(病情轻重、有无合并症、诊断经过等),受试对象及对照者的来源、正常值如何规定、该诊断方法如何具体进行等。②研究疾病的临床经过及预后的论文:要注意说明患者是在病程的哪个阶段接受治疗、患者的转诊情况,观察疾病结果的客观指标等。③病因学研究论文:需说明所研究设计方法(如临床随机试验、队列研究等)、是否做了剂量-效应观察等。④对临床疗效观察的研究:主要说明病例选择的标准、病例的一般资料(性别、年龄、病情轻重等)、分组原则与样本分配方法(配对、配伍等)、疗效观察指标及标准等。⑤治疗方法的论文:如是手术,则应注明手术名称、术式、麻醉方法等;如是药物治疗,则应注明药物的名称、来源(批号)、剂量、给药途径、疗程,草药还应说明产地及制备方法等。

例 1 From July 2003 to September 2004, we enrolled 428 children into a randomized, double blind trial of three different daily micronutrient supplementation regimens given from 6–24 months of age. The main study outcomes were prevalent days of diarrhea, with secondary outcomes being other diarrhea measures, respiratory morbidity, and growth. The study was done at the Africa Center for Health and Population Studies(AC), which is located in northern rural KwaZulu-Natal

Province, South Africa. The study area has unemployment rates of more than 50%, agriculture underdevelopment, and high HIV prevalence, reaching a peak of 52% for women of 25–29 years. It is a rural area with only one recently tarred road. Study staff consisted of 4 nurses, 17 field workers, 4 supervisors, and a field worker coordinator, all of whom were locally hired. All had at least 5 years of secondary school education but little or no research experience. Ethical approval was granted by the University of Natal Ethics Committee (Durban) and the Tuff-New-England IRB (Boston).

（2）动物：使用动物作为研究对象时，需要把动物的性别、年龄、数量、体重、物种、品种、生理状况、来源、饲养条件、饲养情况、护理条件，以及是否符合国际上拟定的动物公约等作一一介绍。动物的年龄可用天、周、月、年为单位，给出绝对值或范围。动物的体重则可用平均值加减标准误或范围来表达。

例 2 **Experimental animals** ICR mice (20–25g) were used in all experiments. The number of mice used for experiments was from 8 to 10 per group. An equal number of mice of both sexes were used; because no sex difference was observed, data from both sexes were pooled for all reported analyses. Mice were purchased from the Dea-Han animal breeding center (Cheongju, Korea). Animals were maintained in a temperature-controlled environment (22℃ ± 2℃), on a 12：12 h light-dark cycle. Mice were given ad libitum assess to food and tap water.

（3）细胞：实验如使用细胞系，则需说明细胞的来源、类别、产地、厂家及培养条件（包括培养液和培养温度）等。

例 3 Human colorectal SW 480 cancer cell line (ATCC, Manassas, VA) was maintained in Leibovitz's L-15 medium with 10% L-glutamine (Gibco, NY), supplemented with 10% fetal bovine serum and penicillin-streptomycin (50 units/ml, Invitrogen, CA), in a humidified incubator (5% CO_2 in air at 37℃) with medium change every 2–3 days. When the cells reach 70%–80% confluency, they were trypsinized, harvested, and seeded into a new tissue culture dish (100mm in diameter).

2. 随机分组方法（Methods of Any Random Assignment of Subjects to Groups） 随机分组方法确保对比组之间基线均衡可比，被认为是减少两组患者选择偏倚的最佳方法。因此，有学者认为正是由于随机分组方法，使得随机对照试验在提高医疗卫生服务中起着至关重要的作用。在临床研究中，正确地实施真正的随机分组是临床试验的关键。成功地实施随机分组依赖于两个相关的步骤：①产生随机分组序列并应用于试验组和对照组。②随机分组方案在随机分组中的隐匿（allocation concealment）。没有隐匿的随机临床试验也称为开放式的随机对照试验。具体要求如下：

（1）如果使用动物进行试验，需要分别介绍动物的详细分组情况。

例 4 The animal study was conducted under aseptic conditions using a rat model (4-week-old male Wistar). In total, 30 rats divided into three groups (ECM/control, ECM/bFGF, and ECM/Re) were used in the study. Rats were anesthetized by intramuscular injection of sodium pentobarbital (30mg/ml). Two test samples of the same type were separately implanted subcutaneously in each rat. The implanted samples were retrieved at 1 week and 1 month (*n*=5 at each time point) postoperatively. At retrieval, the appearance of each retrieved sample was examined grossly and photographed. Subsequently, one half of each retrieved sample was fixed and embedded in paraffin for histologic examinations, and the remainder was used to qualify the amount of tissue hemoglobin and to measure denaturation temperature.

（2）如果使用细胞进行实验，也必须把细胞的类型、数量、传代次数、具体分组情况，以及具体实验测定方法进行全面细致的说明。

例 5 To evaluate the *in vitro* expression of IL-6 by human ovarian cancer cell lines, 2×10^5 cells were seeded into individual wells of a six-well plate. Following a 24-hour incubation, cells were washed with PBS, and 1ml of 10% FBS/DMEM was added to each well. After 48 hours, tumor cell-conditioned medium was collected, centrifuged to pellet any detached cells and tested for the presence of human IL-6 by ELISA（R&D System）. To evaluate the expression of soluble IL-6R by human ovarian cancer cell lines, 1×10^5 cells were seeded into individual wells of a 24-well plate and incubated overnight. Cells were then washed with PBS and 0.3ml of 10% FBS/DMEM was added to each well. After 72 hours, tumor cell-conditioned medium was collected, centrifuged to pellet any detached cells, and tested for the presence of the soluble IL-6R by ELISA（R&D System）.

3. 试验所用的药物 试验中所使用的药物、化学药品、试剂等必须注明名称、商标、生产厂家、纯度、浓度、出产公司、产地、城市和国别等。

例 6 ...the following criteria were used for acceptance of an analytical run: the standard curve composed of eight different concentrations must have a $r^2 \geq 0.98$, the A_{450} from the highest concentration must be ≥ 1.5, 4 of 6 positive controls must be detected within $\pm 25\%$ of the expected values, the A_{450} from the negative control must be ≤ 0.5, and the coefficient of variation for each point must be $\leq 25\%$...

4. 试验设备 试验中所使用的仪器、设备和装置均需要说明名称、型号、商标、生产厂家或公司、产地等。

例 7 ...Particles were examined with a FEI Tecnai F30 electron microscope（FEI Company, Hillaboro, OR）. OpenLab software version 3.1.5（Improvision Inc., Lexington, MA）was used in the measurement of particle size.

5. 统计学分析处理 统计学处理是该部分中必不可少的内容，在这一部分，需要说明三方面的数据处理方法。

（1）所使用的统计学方法，如 Paired/Unpaired Student's *t* test、ANOVA 等，不必介绍进行统计学处理的具体过程及程序。

（2）数据的表示方法，是使用平均值 ± 标准差，还是使用平均值 ± 标准误都需要具体说明。在实际的写作过程中，还需要根据目标杂志的要求来确定。

（3）说明在统计过程中所使用的 *P* 值的标准。

例 8 The between-men differences were analyzed using StatView statistical software（Abacus Concepts）. The results were expressed as the mean ± SD of four determinations made in three different experiments, and the differences determined using the two-tailed Student's *t*-test for paired samples. Values of P<5% were considered statistically significant. Differences in cytolytic effects produced by effector CTLs were evaluated taking into account the percentage of specific cytotoxicity at all effector/target cell ratios. Therefore, P values were calculated using covariance analysis performed on the regression of the percentage of specific Cr-release over the logarithm of the number of effector cells/well. All data relative to cell-mediated cytolysis are expressed in terms of mean LU50/106 values without conventional SE or SD of the mean. Actually no statistical analysis can be performed using these parameters, which are not suitable for covariance analysis for regression lines.

三、英文写作中的常用句式

(一) 研究对象的选择、来源及标准

研究对象通常指患者(patients)、受试者(subjects)、健康志愿者(healthy volunteers)、动物(animals)。

1. 纳入研究

(1) ...were entered into/recruited from/enrolled in/selected randomly from...

(2) The major criteria for inclusion in the study were...

(3) To be eligible for the study, ...were required to...

(4) Inclusion/Entry criteria consisted of/were...

(5) Selection was based on...

(6) ...were selected based on...

(7) ...were defined as...

2. 排除或退出研究

(1) Exclusion criteria included...

(2) ...be excluded from participation/enrollment/the study if...

(3) ...be excluded if they had any of the following...

(4) ...be considered ineligible for the following reasons...

(5) ...withdraw from the study due to/because of...

例9　A total of 169 patients were included in the study, 83 of whom received trimetazidine orally at an initial dose of 60mg followed by 20mg tid for 5 days. These patients formed the study group while the remaining 86, the control group.

例10　Twenty-seven patients over age 65, with left ventricular systolic dysfunction, were age-and-sex-matched with 19 patients with normal left ventricular systolic function. Patients with significant mitral or aortic valvular diseases were excluded.

(二) 研究对象的分组及标准

1. ...were divided/stratified/allocated/classified/assigned/grouped into...

2. ...were divided into...based on/on the basis of/depending on...

3. ...were divided randomly/randomized/equally into...

例 11　Based on gestational age, 32 normal primigravid patients were divided into three groups: Group I (*n*=11), less than 12 gestational weeks; group II (*n*=10), 13 to 26 gestational weeks, and group III (*n*=11), 27 gestational weeks or more.

例 12　To clarify these issues, we randomized 70 patients undergoing aortic valve replacement to an aortic hemorrhage group (group A=37 patients; 53%; 34 males, 3 females) and a pulmonary autograft group (group B=33 patients; 47%; 28 males, 5 females).

（三）年龄

1. 达到某一年龄, 如一个 50 岁的患者：

（1）a 50-year-old patient

（2）a patient aged 50 years

（3）a patient at 50 years of age

（4）a patient at the age of 50 years (**NOT**: a patient at the age of 50 years old)

（5）patients (age 50 ± 3 years)

2. 在某年龄段范围内及平均年龄：

（1）(patients) range in age from...to..., with a mean of 50 years

（2）(patients) ranging in age from...to..., with a mean of 50 years

（3）(patients) having an age range of...to... (mean 50 years)

（4）(patients) with a mean/an average age of 50 years (range 35 to 74)

（5）(patients) aged 40 to 50 years

3. 在某一年龄以上或以下：

（1）(patients) 50 years and/or older

（2）(patients) more than/over 50 years

（3）(patients) under/below/less than 50 years

例 13　Ages of these patients ranged/varied from 12 to 65 years (mean 39 ± 15 years) for group A and from 3 to 54 years (mean 29 ± 15 years) for group B.

例 14　The authors examined a stratified random sample of 2,243 men and women aged 45–64 years (mean, 51.3), of whom 260 had myocardial infarction and 1,983 were free of any coronary heart disease manifestations.

（四）性别

1. 12 patients (7 male and 5 female)

2. SD rats of both sexes

3. mixed-bred dogs or either sex

4. The male-to-female ratio was...

例 15　The male-to-female ratio was 1 : 4. The mean age at onset was 11.5 years (range 7–16 years) and the mean duration of disease was 6.5 years (range 3–13 years).

（五）实验方法

be investigated/measured/diagnosed/assessed/examined/treated using/by/with

例 16 Data on 70 burn patients aged 60 years or more who were treated at a regional burn center were analyzed using both univariate and multivariate methods.

例 17 Wound healing was assessed by measurement of changes in mechanical strength and collagen deposition.

（六）实验动物

实验研究论文中，应说明采用何种实验动物，动物的年龄、体重、性别、来源、饲养条件和动物模型饲养方法等。

1. 来源一般在括号内简单说明即可，也可用以下句型表达：

（1）be purchased/obtained from...

（2）be provided by...

（3）be a gift of/from...

（4）be generously donated by...

2. 饲养条件

（1）be bred in...

（2）be fed/maintained with...

（3）be caged individually, fed ad libitum with tap water and...diet

（4）be maintained/raised under...

（5）be fasted/starved 12h prior to operation

3. 处死方法

（1）be sacrificed by decapitation/cervical dislocation

（2）be sacrificed by exsanguination/be exsanguinated

（3）be sacrificed 2h before the experiment

例 18 Animals were maintained in a temperature-controlled environment (22℃ ± 2℃), on a 12 : 12h light-dark cycle. Mice were given ad libitum assess to food and tap water.

（七）借鉴他人实验方法

研究中所用的方法若是借鉴他人的，文中不必详细描述方法过程，但要说明是谁的方法及出处。

1. be done according to the method/technique described previously by...

2. be done/carried out as previously described/in the literature

3. be done/estimated as detailed elsewhere

4. be done with a modified method of...

5. be isolated by the procedure of...

6. be prepared according to the method described by...

7. be separated by the technique described previously...

8. be determined as described except that....

9. Our technique was similar to that of..., except that...

10. The essay was essentially the same as described by...except that...

（八）诊断与治疗

1. 诊断

（1）（patients）be diagnosed as having.../be diagnosed as...by.../with.../according to the basis of...

（2）（patients）be misdiagnosed as having.../be misdiagnosed as...

（3）be mistaken for...

（4）be suspected as.../of having.../to be...

2. 治疗

（1）be treated with...（alone or in combination with...）

（2）（treatment）be initiated/started/discontinued/interrupted/withdrawn/completed

（3）be on（a therapy, e. g. a diet/radiotherapy/chemotherapy/drops...）

（4）be treated on an outpatient/inpatient basis

（5）be referred/transferred to...

练习

1. 根据所给汉语提示完成句子。

（1）Unless noted otherwise, all tissue culture media and supplements _____
_____（从……购买）Invitrogen. Human cervical carcinoma（C-33A）cell line
_____（从……获得）American Tissue Culture Collection（ATCC HTB-31）.

（2）To screen for autoimmunity, all patients before therapy received an ophthalmologic
examination that was repeated _____（三个月后）on study. At baseline patients
were negative for serum thyroglobulin Ab, rheumatoid factor, and antinuclear Ab; while on
study, human anti-human（anti-idiotypic）Ab, erythrocyte sedimentation rate, antinuclear Ab,
thyroid-stimulating hormone, and free T4 were tested _____（每三周）.

（3）_____（麻醉的）female Wistar rats, 240-320g body weight（Charles
River-Wiga, Sulzfeld, Germany）were used for the determination of the elimination half life
of selected inhibitors, _____（如前所述）.

（4）Approximately 8 weeks before admission, the patient was seen in the emergency room
of a local hospital because of respiratory symptoms. Clarithromycin _____
（给她开了克拉霉素）, but the symptoms worsened.

（5）From 2000 to 2004, 97 cases _____（70 岁以上）with cholelithiasis
were retrospectively analyzed. _____（男女患者比例）is 1 : 72.

2. 汉译英。

（1）在第1、3、5、7、9、11、13天分别截图,并传输至私人电脑进行图像分析,如下所述。

（2）以危害比（hazard ratio）及其95%的可信区间（confidence interval）对治疗效果进行衡量,并使用Cox比例风险模型（Cox proportional-hazards model）对治疗效果加以评估。

（3）研究选取稳定型冠心病患者为受试对象。附录详细介绍了入选和排除标准。入选的患者在签署知情同意书之后将接受随机分组。

（4）936名男性患者的平均年龄为48.5岁（7~96岁）,404名女性患者的平均年龄为49.6岁（10~78岁）。

（5）依照欧洲呼吸协会的推荐采用了痰诱导（sputum induction）的方法,用二硫赤藓糖醇（dithioerythritol）迅速处理标本,从痰液相（fluid phase of sputum）中分离出细胞。

（鲍霞）

第七节　结　果

一、综述

结果（results）是医学科技论文的根基、核心和重要组成部分,因为这部分内容包含了支持论文中提出的观点或假设的全部资料。从根本上说,一篇论文的水平高低取决于结果的价值。无论人们是否把结果放在首位来阅读,结果在论文中的作用都极为重要,不可忽视。

在结果部分,作者需要回答这样一个问题:在研究中观察到什么现象（What did you observe）。可见,论文中撰写"结果"有两个目的:

（1）告诉读者在研究期间发生了什么（to tell what happened during the study）。一般而言,为引起读者注意,作者应当最先介绍最重要的结果。

（2）展示研究中的发现（to present the findings of the study）。这就要求作者把所观察到的结果,客观而准确地呈现在读者面前。经过组织、总结、分析、科学归纳及统计学处理,采用文字和图表兼用的方式,把在实验中所观察到的现象、所记录的数据、所拍摄的资料和所测试的数据等清楚地呈现在结果部分。

二、写作要求

结果部分为读者展示材料与方法部分所述主要实验的主要结果。因此,打算参考论文实验方法的读者,一定会同时参考其材料与方法和结果部分,从而对自己拟开展的相关实验可能得出的结果有所预测。同时,重点关注论文主要结论的读者,也会参考结果和讨论部

分,以便对论文的学术价值做出判断。撰写结果部分时,需要注意以下问题:

1. 本部分的基本时态是过去时。

2. 为使行文更具整体感,本部分可概述上文(引言或材料与方法部分)出现过的要点,但不要赘述细节。

3. 列举出最能体现研究结果的代表性数据,而不是将研究得出的数据不加选择地全部列出。对数据的评论则应集中在讨论部分进行。

4. 在表述结果的统计学意义时,避免使用诸如 highly、nearly 等程度副词修饰 significant。

5. 利用图和表简化本部分的文字叙述。

6. 提及阴性的实验结果时,一般不需要给出具体数据。

三、写作形式

(一) 适合用文字表达的情况

在实际的论文撰写过程中,并不是所有的数据或结果都可以在图表中展示,还需要经常在正文中进行文字表述。这些数据可以简洁和清楚地用文字加以说明。以下情况适于用文字表达:

1. 结果中数据的数量较少,能做同类比较的观测项目不多,可以直接用文字表达,不必用图或表来表述。

2. 结果的因素单一,与实验中的其他资料无法联系或没有太大关系的数据,一般不宜或无法用图表来表达。

3. 以观察形态特征为主的论文,一般不适于用表格表达,而以文字表述为主,配合形态学图片。

例 1 Quantitative analysis using HPLC method showed that the content of ginsenoside Re was 99.3%, indicating that the Re sample used in this study was high purity.

例 2 Seed production was higher for plants in the full-sun treatment (52.3 ± 6.8) than for those receiving filtered light $(14.7 \pm 3.2, P<0.001)$.

例 3 In all 11 cases, viable tumor tissue grafts were obtained under kidney capsules of female NOD/SCID mice, as indicated by H&E staining of section. Growth of the xenografts was slow, except for the grade 3 transitional/undifferentiated cancer that grow twice as much volume within 15 days. No metastasis was observed in any of the hosts during the study period. Of a total of 108 tissue implantations, 104 were successful, resulting in an overall engraftment rate>95%.

(二) 图和表在论文中的运用

在科技论文中,插图是一种形象化的表达方式,而表格是简明的、规范化的科学用语。图表在论文的表达中确实发挥相当重要的作用。归纳起来有:①展示数据并说明数据变化;②对实验数据进行直观比较;③有效而形象地表达结果;④简化文字,提高论文清晰度;⑤展示原始数据记录。

设计图表的基本要求可概括为:正确合理、简明清晰,且具有"自明性"(self-explanatoriness)。

自明性是指通过图和表就能大体了解研究的基本结果和内容,是衡量图表的重要标志。使用图和表时要注意以下几点:

1. 结果部分插入的图和表应该精选,体现科研论文行文简明的特点。

2. 按照图和表在结果部分出现的顺序分别对其进行相应的编号。

3. 设计的图和表应具有自明性,使读者不用参考正文文字就可理解图和表的内容。

4. 表的上方应该有标题,而图注应在图的下方。标题和图注应该言简意赅,避免结果部分正文和表图之间的重复、赘述。例如:

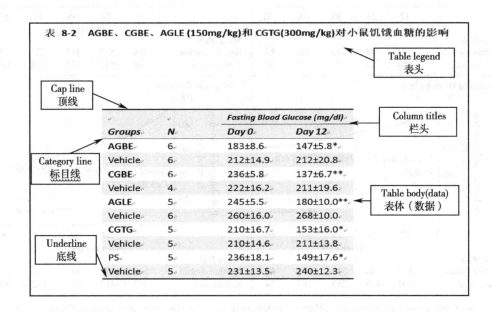

表 8-2 AGBE、CGBE、AGLE (150mg/kg)和 CGTG(300mg/kg)对小鼠饥饿血糖的影响

Groups	N	Fasting Blood Glucose (mg/dl)	
		Day 0	Day 12
AGBE	6	183±8.6	147±5.8*
Vehicle	6	212±14.9	212±20.8
CGBE	6	236±5.8	137±6.7**
Vehicle	4	222±16.2	211±19.6
AGLE	5	245±5.5	180±10.0**
Vehicle	6	260±16.0	268±10.0
CGTG	5	210±16.7	153±16.0*
Vehicle	5	210±14.6	211±13.8
PS	5	236±18.1	149±17.6*
Vehicle	5	231±13.5	240±12.3

* $P<0.05$
** $P<0.01$ compared to vehicle group
AGBE: American ginseng berry extract.
CGBE: Chinese ginseng berry extract.
AGLE: American ginseng leaf extract.
CGTG: Total ginsenosides in Chinese Ginseng
PS: Polysaccharide.

(三) 表头和图注的表示方法

虽然不同的杂志对表头和图注的表示方法没有统一的规定和字数的限制,一般来说,在撰写论文时还是要注意以下几点:

1. 图注和表头必须清楚而准确地表达图表的内容。

2. 图注和表头不一定是一个完整的句子,可以由一些词、词组及动名词组成,其文字应力求简明,做到用最少的文字表达准确而清楚的含义。例如:

Table 1 Patients' age, tumor histopathology and stage

3. 在图注之后,还有必要进一步说明,这些说明性文字则必须使用完整的句子。例如:

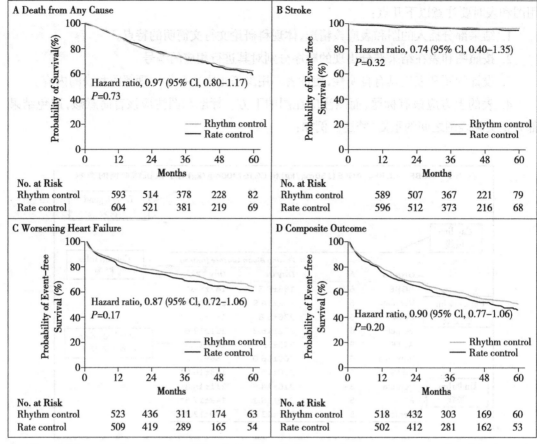

Figure 3:Kaplan-Meier Estimates of Secondary Outcomes

None of the secondary outcomes differed significantly between the treatment groups. Panel A shows the probability of death from any cause(32% in the rhythm-control group and 33% in the rate-control group),Panel B shows the probability of ischemic or hemorrhagic stroke(3% and 4%,respectively),Panel C...There were also no significant differences favoring either strategy in any of the predefined subgroups. Hazard ratios are for the rhythm-control group,as compared with the rate-control group.

（四）图表在正文中的提出

写作论文时,有一个不成文的规定,就是在展示或说明每一个图表之前,必须首先在文中提出来,而后才加以分析、解释、注释和使用。常见的方法有以下几种:

1. 开门见山式,即直接在文中提出图名或表名,并详细剖析图或表的内容。

例 4　Figure 2 shows three sets of microscopic currents recorded on excised inside-out patches from oocytes expressing wild-type Kir 2.1 channels.

例 5　Results of this analysis are presented in Table 5 and in Figures 2,3,4 and 5.

由于图和表是为作者的观点提供支撑材料和数据,因此在结果正文部分中提及图和表时,不宜将其作为句子的主语。显然,例 5 在表述上优于例 4。

2. 描述内容式,即先概括描述图或表的主要内容,其后用圆括号引出图或表。

例 6　In line with our previous experience for benign tissues,the sub-renal capsule site was found to be extremely efficient with nearly 95% of grafts recovered（Table 1）.

3. 其他引导形式，比如用短语引出图或表，随后再加上必要的文字说明。

例 7　As shown in Figure 3B, cell death increased significantly after H_2O_2 exposure from $(5.0 \pm 1.6)\%$ to $(52.1 \pm 3.0)\%$ $(n=10, P<0.001)$.

四、英文写作中的常用句式

1. 结果表明……

（1）The results showed/demonstrated/revealed/documented/indicated/
　　　suggested/displayed that...

（2）The results failed to show/confirm/support...

（3）It was found that...

（4）We found that...

（5）...was/were found to...

例 8　These results indicated that a substantial fraction of the most strongly associated single-nucleotide polymorphisms（单核苷酸多态性）could have true associations with bone mineral density.

2. 研究对象的分组、随机及去向：

（1）...were randomized into

（2）...were randomly divided/allocated/categorized/assigned into...

例 9　In a phase 2, double bind, 48-week trial involving 104 patients with relapsing-remitting multiple sclerosis, we assigned 69 patients to receive 1,000mg of intravenous rituximab and 35 patients to receive placebo on days 1 and 15.

例 10　Of 7,428 patients who underwent screening, 4,458 were randomly assigned to study groups.

例 11　A total of 4,761 patients entered the placebo run-in phase. Of these, 3,845 were randomly assigned to one of the two study groups.

例 12　The numbers of participants who were assessed for safety were 2,220 in the rosiglitazone group and 2,227 in the control group.

例 13　We randomly assigned 751 women with gestational diabetes mellitus at 20 to 33 weeks of gestation to open treatment with metformin（with supplemental insulin if required）or insulin.

例 14　The exclusion criteria were a prepregnancy diagnosis of diabetes, a contraindication to metformin, a fetal anomaly, gestational hypertension, preeclampsia, fetal growth restriction, and ruptured membranes.

例 15　Randomization was performed with a block size of four and was stratified according to site and gestational age（from 20 weeks to 27 weeks and 6 days, or from 28 weeks to 33 weeks and 6 days）.

3. 与……有关 / 无关

（1）A was（not）related/correlated/associated with B

（2）There was（not）a relationship/correlation/association between A and B

（3）There was（not）a relationship/correlation of A with B and C

（4）A was（not）in relation/correlation/association to B

（5）A was（not）found to be related/correlated/associated with B

（6）We found（no）clear relationship/difference between...and...

（7）The dose-response relationship appeared to be slightly stronger for...

（8）A was（not）involved/implicated in B

部分形容词或副词可以用在以上句型中起修饰作用，如 significant（ly），strong（ly），inverse（ly），negative（ly），positive（ly），indirect（ly），linear，proportional。

例 16 Log-rank analysis identified expression of both CD90 and EpCAM was significantly associated with survival time of HCC patients.

例 17 Fetal head is proportional to vertebral column under normal condition；CSD correlates well with BPD（$r=0.982\,7$，$P<0.001$）. The regression formula was CSD=6.45+1.53 BPD.

4. 增加或减少

（1）从……增加到……，平均增加……

to increase from...to..., with an average/a mean increase of...

（2）从……增加到……，总的增加……

to increase from...to..., with an overall increase of...

（3）增加到 10%：to increase to（10%）

（4）增加了 10%：to increase by（10%）/to increase（10%）/a（10%）increase in...

5. 倍数比较

（1）增加或减少（3 倍）

to increase/decrease by 3 fold/times

a 3-fold increase/decrease

（2）A 是 B 的 3 倍

A is 3 fold/times as...as B

A is 3 fold/times B

6. 结果的统计学意义

（1）There was/is significant difference in...between A and B

（2）The difference in...between A and B was/is significant.

（3）A was/is significantly different from B in...

（4）A was significantly different from the control value，$P<0.01$.

（5）No significant difference was found/observed/noted in...between A and B（in 后面接区分的性质或内容）

例 18 There was no statistically significant difference between Group A and Group B.

例 19 Patients in Group A had a significantly higher risk of congestive heart failure than did patients in the control group, with 38 versus 17 adjudicated events (hazard ratio, 2.24; 95% CI, 1.27 to 3.97).

例 20　A higher proportion of men was present in control group 1 than in the mitotane（米托坦，抗肿瘤药）group（$P=0.05$），whereas sex distribution in control group 2 did not differ significantly from that in the mitotane group.

例 21　Differences between the two groups remained significant（$P=0.04$；odds ratio, 1.8; 95% CI, 1.0 to 3.2）

7. 描述不良反应

（1）...discountinued the study drug because...developed.

（2）No serious events were identified..., but...were detected...

（3）...was reported as a complication of...

（4）The treatment-related adverse events were...

例 22　One patient in the amphotericin group discontinued the study drug after receiving 8 doses because pulmonary tuberculosis developed.

例 23　No serious events were identified during the test sessions, but in four participants, serious medical conditions were detected 1 to 30 days later.

例 24　Hypotension was reported as a complication of therapy during 18.5% of intermittent hemodialysis sessions in the intensive strategy as compared with 18.9% in the less-intensive strategy.

例 25　The most frequent treatment-related adverse events were headache and abdominal pain. There were no significant cardiovascular effects of treatment.

例 26　Acute mountain sickness occurred in 7.4% of the participants, but its frequency did not vary significantly among the altitudes studied.

8. versus/vs./v. 表示数值对比

当几组数值进行比较时，完全用文字表达不仅篇幅累赘，也难以让读者一目了然。可以使用 versus, vs. 或 v. 形式来表达。

例 27　Anticoagulation with bivalirudin alone, as compared with heparin plus glycoprotein Ⅱ b/Ⅲ a inhibitors, resulted in a reduced 30-day rate of net adverse clinical events（9.2% vs. 12.1%；relative risk, 0.76; 95% CI, 0.63 to 0.92; $P=0.005$），owing to a lower rate of major bleeding（4.9% vs. 8.3%；relative risk, 0.60; 95% CI, 0.46 to 0.77; $P<0.001$）.

9. 描述患者跟踪调查

（1）The median duration of follow-up was...

（2）Treatment was continued until...

（3）...were still in follow-up.

（4）...were lost to follow-up.

例 28　Approximately 10% of patients（218 in the rosiglitazone group and 223 in the control group）were lost to follow-up.

例 29　No subjects were lost to follow-up.

例 30 Eleven other participants withdrew voluntarily during the study: 8 because of symptoms of discomfort and 3 for personal reasons.

例 31 In total, 675 patients (263 in the rosiglitazone group and 412 in the control group) withdrew from receiving study drugs but were still in follow-up.

例 32 The median duration of follow-up was 1.8 years (mean, 2.1; range, 0 to 6.5).

例 33 Treatment was continued until June 2006, and follow-up ended in January 2007.

10. 其他表达方式

A 与 B 相似:A is similar to/analogous to B

相反:in contrast/by contrast/on the contrary/whereas

与……一致:be consistent with/the same as/be comparable with (to)…

　　　　　We found a marked similarity between...and...

就……而言 / 在……方面:with respect to/with regard to...

不论其……:regardless of...

以……表示:be present as...

A 越……B 越……(表示一个指标随另一个指标变化而变化):The longer the..., the faster the...

例 34 Sensitivity analyses showed that the proportional contributions of specific treatments and risk-factor changes to the overall reduction in deaths from coronary heart disease in 2000 were relatively consistent.

例 35 In contrast, the increase in the body-mass index (the weight in kilograms divided by the square of the height in meters) of 2.6 and the 2.9% increase in the prevalence of diabetes resulted in...

例 36 By contrast, the endoplasmic reticulum was detectable in both the inner and the peripheral cytoplasmic zones.

例 37 Mortality was similar between the two treatment groups with regard to all prespecified subgroups.

例 38 The lower the gestational age of the index participant, the greater the risk of having less than a high school education and the lower the risk of having graduate education.

练习

1. 根据所给汉语提示完成句子。

(1) To assess the relative contribution of genes to the variance in YKL-40 levels among subjects, we first estimated the heritability of the YKL-40 level. The high estimate for broad heritability ＿＿＿＿＿＿＿＿＿＿(说明 / 表明 / 提示 / 暗示) that differences in serum YKL-40 levels among individual Hutterites ＿＿＿＿＿＿＿＿＿＿(几乎完全是因为) genetic differences between individual persons.

（2）The mean gestational age at delivery（分娩平均妊娠年龄）for the metformin group and the insulin group was 38.3 weeks and 38.5 weeks, ＿＿＿＿＿＿＿＿＿＿＿＿（分别地）. There was ＿＿＿＿＿＿＿＿＿＿＿＿＿＿（统计学上显著但在临床上细微的差异）.

（3）＿＿＿＿＿＿＿＿＿＿＿＿＿＿（治疗过程中突然出现的不良事件）were reported by 166 of the 207 patients（80.2%）receiving 2mg of prucalopride, 160 of the 204 patients（78.4%）receiving 4mg of prucalopride, and 149 of the 209 patients（71.3%）receiving placebo. ＿＿＿＿＿＿＿＿＿＿＿＿＿＿（最常见报道的药物不良反应）were headache, nausea, abdominal pain, and diarrhea.

（4）＿＿＿＿＿＿＿＿＿＿＿＿＿＿（没有显著效果）of the type of glucose control on major macrovascular events, death from cardiovascular causes, or death from an cause（hazard ratio with intensive control, 0.93; 95% CI, 0.83 to 1.06; $P=0.28$）.

（5）Changes in medical treatments ＿＿＿＿＿＿＿（占）approximately 47% and risk-factor changes ＿＿＿＿＿＿（占）approximately 44% of the decrease in deaths.

2. 汉译英。

（1）经过平均5年的随访，强化治疗组（6.5%）的平均糖化血红蛋白（glycated hemoglobin）水平低于标准控制组（或非强化治疗组）（7.3%）。

（2）分娩后（post partum）6~8周，552（75.3%）位产妇进行了75克口服糖耐量测试（oral glucose-tolerance test）。270名二甲双胍组中有62名（23.0%）和282名胰岛素组中58名（20.6%）糖耐量受损或被诊断为糖尿病。

（3）在二甲双胍组和胰岛素组间，分娩时的平均妊娠年龄（38.3周 vs. 38.5周）存在统计学上显著但是临床上细微的差异。

（4）特比萘分（terbinafine）耐受性好，副作用轻至中度，且常为一过性（transient）的。最常见的有胃肠道症状（胀满感、食欲不振、恶心、轻度腹痛或腹泻）或轻微的皮肤反应（皮疹、荨麻疹等）。

（5）三人死于与肾病无关的原因。在其余20个患者中，52%的患者其肾功能保持稳定至少2年之久。在随访2年以上的9个患者中，4人复发，但再次治疗全部有效。没有发现预示复发的特别临床症状，尽管所有患者都出现血尿（hematuria）和蛋白尿（proteinuria）。治疗的并发症较为常见，这可能是造成两名患者死亡的原因。

（宋红波）

第八节　讨　论

讨论（discussion）是顺承结果部分的重要环节，是一篇论文的灵魂所在。这一部分最能反映作者对相关文献的阅读量以及对某个学术问题理解的深度和广度。因此，这一部分是医学英文论文写作中较为困难的一个环节。在讨论中,作者围绕着研究发现、实验结果、最新理论基础、未来研究设想等核心问题,进一步提炼和升华研究意义和价值,将对实验结果表现的感性认识上升为理性认识。通过讨论,读者可以了解到该论文的理论意义和实际应用价值以及该论文是否可以扩展到其他领域或是否有助于理解更广泛的领域。总之,讨论是一篇论文中"讲道理"的部分,作者应把所要阐述的道理、机制、事物内部的深层联系及可能的规律在这里说清楚。这样可以帮助读者更好地理解和消化吸收研究结果,有助于科研成果的交流与传播。如果说读者是通过一篇论文的摘要部分而选择是否要阅读该篇论文的话,那么讨论部分往往决定了该篇论文是否能够发表。因此,讨论的好与坏,对于一篇论文至关重要。

一、讨论的内容

1. 回答引言提出的问题,概述研究的主要发现。在讨论的开头应开门见山地给出研究结果,无需引用数据或研究设计。

例 1 **In this study, we have shown that** tumor cells organize a mitochondrial chaperone network, which involves Hsp90, its related molecule, TRAP-1, and the immunophilin CypD. This complex maintains mitochondrial homeostasis and antagonizes the function of CypD in permeability transition. Conversely, inhibition of mitochondrial Hsp90 chaperones with a novel class of mitochondria-directed ATPase antagonists causes sudden loss of mitochondrial membrane potential, release of cytochrome c, and massive death of tumor but not normal cells.

2. 指出本研究结果与其他学者的研究结果的异同,进行文献综述,重点说明本文的创新点和对创新点的支撑。

例 2 **In previous studies,** the antitumor effect of HNP1 was identified primarily with purified HNP1 protein *in vitro* but has not been well explored *in vivo* mainly due to the lack of efficient manufacture of mature HNP1 peptide and, more importantly, due to the inhibition to cytotoxicity of HNP1 through serum proteins. **The present studies show** that cancer gene therapy by the intratumoral delivery of plasmid DNA encoding HNP1 could effectively inhibit tumor growth in A549 xenograft model. The antitumor effect depends on the intracellular expression of *HNP1*, which directly induces apoptosis in tumor cells, and might involve anti-angiogenesis through locally secreted HNP1. The results suggest that gene therapy with de novo expression of *HNP1*, by introducing mature peptide *in vivo*, could provide an attractive alternative.

In contrast to other data (Ref), we show that Shh is sufficient to increase the number of neurospheres derived from SVZ cultures grown over quiescent astrocytes. **This difference might relate to the method used:** it is possible that the astrocytes in the feeder layer produce enough cofactors but at low enough levels for Shh to act, whereas saturating levels of EGF mask the effects of Shh (Ref).

3. 说明或解释结果,用假设理论来解释试验中非常新的东西,做到自圆其说,同时根据这些结果,阐述本研究的结论。

例 3 The antidiabetic effect of ginseng root has recently been demonstrated. For instance, Kimura *et al* observed a notable fall in blood glucose levels 6 h after a single 90mg/kg ginseng root extract IP dose in genetically obese diabetic KK-CAy mice. **However, when studying a chronic disease such as diabetes, it is more pertinent to test the maintenance of lower blood glucose levels with long-term treatment rather than the acute hypoglycemic effect after a single dose. In this study, we measured** fasting blood glucose 5 and 12 days after treatment. Unlike the short-term treatment study, we found that these compounds progressively reduced blood glucose levels in *ob/ob* mice.

4. 分析、解释本研究的不足之处或局限性,提出今后研究的方向与存在的问题。

例 4 The target-aimed biomolecules could promote downregulation of the VEGF reportor-3 signaling pathway or blockade of ligands VEGF-D to prevent any unestablished lymphatic endothelium from sprouting in a similar manner as has been revealed by the immunohistochemistry assay. **However, blocking of VEGF reportor-3 signaling could only suppress tumor lymph angiogenesis and metastases to regional LNs but not to the lungs.** AdIL-12-engineered MSC administration could even reverse metastasis to the lungs besides that of regional LNs; therefore its antimetastasic effects **may be more complicated and go beyond mere interference with the VEGF receptor-3 signaling pathway** as the lymphatic sprout inhibitor. **This aspect is worth exploring in-depth in future study.**

5. 指出结果的理论意义和实际应用,论述研究结果的潜在价值。

例 5 The results presented here **demonstrate** an involvement of Shh signaling in the regulation of SVZ stem cells, leading to sustained neurogenesis, in the postnatal and adult mouse brain. Taken together, the gene expression analyses and the *in vitro* and *in vivo* experiments **indicate** that Shh signaling is critical for the modulation of the number of cells with stem cell properties, for the proliferation of early precursors consequently for the production of new neurons.

In summary, Hsp90-directed protein folding/refolding **functions as** a novel regulatory of mitochondrial permeability transition(reference). Although this pathway is selectively exploited in tumor cells to elevate an antiapoptotic threshold, **the development of Hsp90 antagonists competent to accumulate in mitochondria may provide a new class of potent and selective anticancer agents, potentially devoid of side effects for normal tissues.**

二、讨论的写作要求

讨论主要是对研究结果的解释和推断,并说明该结果是否支持或反对某种观点,并提出新问题或观点等。因此,撰写讨论时,论点要讲清楚,论述要有根据,做到每个结论都要有证据。

1. 讨论应围绕研究结果展开,主次分明。深入探讨重要结果,突出研究的创新性。

2. 多层次多角度讨论问题。

3. 论据要具有说服力和逻辑性。可以从本研究的结果、实验设计和理论原理的角度进行阐述。

4. 观点或结论的表述要清楚明确。结果与讨论前后呼应,相互衬托。

5. 讨论的结尾,要客观评价研究中的局限性,提出今后的研究方向。

6. 客观表述科学意义和实际应用,做到实事求是,并适当留有余地。例如,可选用 prove、demonstrate 等表示作者坚信观点的真实性;选用 show、indicate、find 等陈述事实;选用 imply、suggest 等表示推测;选用情态动词 can、could、may、should、will 等或者副词 probably、possibly 等表示对论点的确定性程度。

三、范文解析

下面以发表在 *Nucleic Acids Research* 的题为 "Real-time expression profiling of microRNA precursors in human cancer cell lines" 的论文的讨论部分(节选)为例,分析讨论部分的写作特点。

(A) Reported here is an extension of our prior real-time PCR assay to include primers to 222 human miRNA precursors. (B) The miRNA precursor expression was profiled in 32 human cancer cell lines. (C) This is the only study to our knowledge to profile miRNA expression in such a large number of cancer cell lines. (D) We also report a novel method to quantify individual members of nearly identical miRNA isoforms using TaqMan MGB probes. (E) The assay was adapted to a 384-well format, allowing for high-throughput quantification of 196 miRNAs in duplicate per reaction plate.

(A) Since the current number of human miRNAs is relatively small (~222) (the number of human miRNAs has increased to 321 since the initial submission of this manuscript), the PCR assay provides a high-throughput screen for most of the miRNA precursors (in duplicate) using a single reaction plate. (B) Other high-throughput assays, such as cDNA microarrays, have been used to profile miRNA expression. (C) The advantage of real-time PCR is that it is more quantitative than cDNA arrays; real-time PCR is able to detect a 2-fold difference in gene expression. (D) The relative sensitivity between cDNA micro arrays and real-time PCR is exemplified by the fact that cDNA microarray expression data is validated by real-time PCR, not the other way around. (E) If the number of human miRNAs remains fairly small, then high-throughput, real-time PCR is a practical means to profile miRNA expression. (F) If the number of human miRNAs increases to 1,000, as recently predicted by Berezikov et al, it will then be possible to profile miRNA expression using PCR; however, it may be less practical than microarrays.

(A) Unsupervised hierarchical clustering of unfiltered data demonstrates that the miRNA expression data produced a near-perfect clustering of the cell lines into the tissue type from which each cell line were ostensibly derived. (B) With the exception of the prostate and breast cancer cell lines, each cell line produced perfect or near-perfect clustering into the respective tissue type. (C) This is remarkable in that the analysis was performed on only 201 genes. (D) Ross et al profiled the expression of 8,000 genes in the 60 cell lines used in the National Cancer Institute screen for anti-cancer drugs. (E) This analysis revealed that each of the cell types produced near-perfect clustering into tissues from which each cell line was derived; some cell lines such as leukemia and colorectal clustered into unique branches while the other 10 lines were split between different trees of the dendrogram. (F) It is interesting that we obtained similar clustering results as Ross et al by profiling only 201 genes compared with 8,000. (G) Explanations include the use of real-time PCR rather than cDNA microarrays and that noncoding miRNAs were profiled rather than protein coding miRNAs. (H) Thus, the idea of a tissue-specific miRNA expression signature may have merit, even among cultured cells. (I) In addition to differences in tissue origin, the cell lines were also from three different cell lineages, epithelial (prostate, breast, colorectal, lung and pancreas), hematopoietic and squamous cell (head and neck). (J) Clustering produced complete separation of the squamous cell and hematopietic cell lines.

(A) Amplification and quantification of the mature miRNA by PCR presents a challenge because the mature miRNA is roughly the size of a standard PCR primer. (B) For this reason, we developed a real-time PCR assay to amplify and quantify the miRNA precursors as a way to predict the levels of the active mature miRNA. (C) Validation of mature miRNA expression was not attempted for each case here; however, validations attempted in this study as well as prior cases by us and others demonstrate that the levels of precursor miRNA often correlate to the mature miRNA. (D) One case for which no correlation exists is the brain-specific miR-9/miR-9. (E) MiR-9 precursors were expressed at very high levels in many of the cell lines; however, we were unable to detect mature miR-9/miR-9 by northern blotting in eight of these cell lines. (F) It will be interesting to see if the processing of miRNA precursors by specific tissues contributes to high levels of certain miRNAs such as miR-9 in brain.

(A) Another issue that has not been thoroughly addressed in the literature is what constitutes "miRNA expression". (B) The difficulty is that northern blotting is currently the gold standard for miRNA detection, yet northern blotting is inherently insensitive. (C) Based upon our extensive analysis of miRNA precursor expression using real-time PCR, we have found that typically only relative precursor expression values>10 are visible by northern blotting (loading 20–30μg total RNA). (D) Approximately 85% of the miRNA precursors studied here had relative expression values<10, so conceivably, many of these mature miRNAs would be undetectable by northern blotting. (E) But does that mean they are not "expressed"? (F) It is also possible that many of the miRNAs appearing as green with relative expression values<0.1 represent background rather than expressed miRNA.

(A) It should be emphasized that the real-time PCR data presented here is for the miRNA precursors and not the active, mature miRNA. (B) The relationship between precursor and mature miRNA expression has not been thoroughly addressed in the literature using sensitive, high-throughput assays. (C) Only until these studies are completed will we have a better understanding of how miRNA processing is regulated in cell lines and in normal and diseased tissues. (D) It is conceivable that the processing of some miRNAs, such as miR-205 and miR-100, are not regulated and that primary transcript levels are processed to mature miRNA in a stoichiometric manner, while others such as miR-9/miR-9 are regulated. (E) Thus, the real-time PCR data presented here should be used as a starting point for those wishing to explore the function of an miRNA in a particular cell line and investigators should begin their study by using northern blotting or perhaps more sensitive assays to ensure that the expression of the mature miRNA is reflected by the precursor expression reported here.

　　本部分共分为六个自然段。第 1 段总结本研究及主要研究结果。第 2~5 段逐条分析与解释本研究及其结果的特色之处。第 6 段得出研究结论,论述本研究的意义。

　　该讨论部分的写作方法和特点如下:

　　第 1 段是对本研究的概括总结,共五个句子。(A) 句和(B) 句对本研究的内容做了总结。(A) 句是一个以 Reported here 开头的倒装句,将表示研究内容的主语后置,避免头重脚轻。(C)~(E) 句从不同角度论述了本研究的先进之处。使用 This is the only study to our knowledge to...、We also report a novel method to... 等句型介绍本研究在同类研究中的领先性。

　　第 2 段将本研究中使用的主要实验方法 PCR assay 与其他方法 cDNA array 进行比较,体现本研究的方法优势。

　　第 3 段将(A)~(C) 句所述实验结果 the miRNA expression data produced a near-perfect clustering of the cell lines into the tissue type from which each cell line were ostensibly derived 与同类研究(D) 句和(E) 句加以比较,得出比较结果(F)。It is interesting that we obtained similar clustering results as Ross et al by profiling only 201 genes compared with 8,000,体现了本研究的优势,即仅用 201 个基因就得出了他人用 8 000 个基因得到的实验结果。(G) 句对这一优势加以解释,(H) 句则推广上述结果,将本研究的结果放到该领域的大背景里加以评价,提出新的观点 Thus, the idea of a tissue-specific miRNA expression signature may have merit, even among cultured cells。(I)~(J) 句评论另一个与此相关但相对次要的研究结果。

　　第 4 段解释本研究选取的实验方案。(A) 句介绍本领域的研究难题 "Amplification and quantification of the mature miRNA by PCR presents a challenge" 并说明原因。(B) 句则说明所选实验方案正是基于上述原因:由于对成熟 miRNA 的 PCR 扩增和定量难以实现,因此本研究以定量 PCR 扩增和定量 miRNA 前体为预测成熟 miRNA 的水平提供依据。(C) 句解答由此产生的问题:miRNA 前体的表达水平能否代表成熟 miRNA 的水平,并证明结果的可信度。(D)~(F) 句解释说明特殊情况,使行文更为严谨。第 4 段进一步论证了本研究的创新性,即巧妙而令人信服地解决了相关领域的一个研究难题。

　　第 5 段以研究涉及的另一个问题 what constitutes "miRNA expression" 为发端,比较了本研究用的基本方法 real-time PCR 和公认的 miRNA 检测的金标准方法 northern blotting 的灵敏度,解答读者可能对本研究产生的质疑,增强本研究结果的说服力。

第6段是讨论部分的结束段,共五个句子,分两层意思。(A)~(D)句论述了本研究的局限性。(E)句则得出论著的结论,"从特异到一般",将研究个体问题得出的结果放到更大的领域中去考量,体现研究的推广价值。作者指出:本研究的结果,即 miRNA 表达的定量 PCR 数据,可以作为研究特定 miRNA 在特定细胞株中的功能的第一步,而后续工作应该从以适当方法验证成熟 miRNA 表达水平与本论文所报道的相应的 miRNA 前体表达水平的一致性开始。

四、注意事项

(一) 避免层次不清,主次不分

泛化的讨论,往往欠缺深入的主题。在讨论中,应紧紧抓住结果中的独特之处。无论问题大小、是否重要,都要从多个角度展开深入讨论,做到有主有次,层次分明。可以通过类比的方法,突显自己结论的创新性。亦可用多种设计方法,深入阐述自己的论文结论与他人的不同之处,从而将重点内容阐述清楚。

(二) 避免重复

这里的避免重复,指的是避免对引言和结果的简单重复。虽然讨论与引言部分援引的问题或假说息息相关,但并不是简单地重复,而是对引言部分从深度和广度上的展开。讨论中涉及结果的话题,要避免过于详细地呈现结果数据,可以借助图表或流程图等方法,原则性和概括性地呈现相关数据。

(三) 避免夸大研究结果的重要性

任何研究均有自身的局限性,在推广应用之前均需要反复的推敲和论证。每一个结果的解释,都需要研究数据的支持。因此,需避免过度夸大研究结果的重要性,否则会引起评审和读者的反感,导致论文被拒。

(四) 避免探讨与实验结果无关或不一致的内容

结果与讨论应该一一对应。避免出现讨论与结果出现不一致或少数讨论的内容可以推出与实验相反的结论的现象。在讨论中,哪怕与结果出现极其细微的差别,也会给人以结果不可信的印象,成为论文被拒的原因。

(五) 避免赘述

讨论中应避免文字冗长、反复叙述、废话过多等现象。虽然国际上一些 SCI 杂志对讨论部分没有明确的字数要求,但撰写讨论时要开门见山、直截了当,给评审和读者以一目了然的印象。

(六) 注意实验数据中的偏差或研究局限

每个研究或论文都有短处或不足,实验中难免存在数据偏差的问题,在讨论中要对数据中的偏差加以说明,增加该实验的客观性和真实性。

(七) 避免夸大、绝对的语言

科技论文完全不同于文学作品,不可使用过分夸张的语言及绝对化的词语。例如,This

therapy will be safely applied to all patients with that disease. 这个句子的表述过于绝对与主观。读者们会质疑,该研究的实验对象是否是该病的全部患者,是否能够找到所有的该病患者。因此,说 all patients 是不符合事实的,过于夸大和绝对。同时,读者们会质疑,该药物是绝对安全的吗? 一般而言,对一种药物来说,安全是有条件的;毒副作用是一定会有的,只不过大小有所不同而已。因此,讲某种药物无任何毒副作用是无根据的,难以确信的。因此,safely 在这里使用不当。

(八) 避免引用文献不足或引用无关文献

在撰写论文时,由于作者对引用相关文献的必要性认识不足或因条件有限,无法查全相关文献,讨论时就会出现文献引用量不够或无法支撑其研究结果等问题,严重影响该论文的创新性和实用价值。

(九) 注意"讨论"的格式

讨论部分无需另外开始新的一页。根据目标杂志的要求,可留有一定的行距和空格,再写上"Discussion"。

五、常用句型总结

1. 总结研究的主要发现,概述最重要的结果

These results suggest/show/indicate that...

In this study, we demonstrate/provide evidence/have found that...

The conclusion that...was drawn from studies on...

We may conclude that...

2. 指出本研究结果与其他学者的研究结果的异同

The first evidence of...comes from...

The findings are further supported by...

This discrepancy may reflect the difference between...and...

3. 说明创新点或创新点论据

This is the only study to our knowledge to...

This study provides the first/direct evidence that...

The major finding of this study is that...

We also reported a novel method to...

4. 说明、解释或猜测结果

We suggest two possible explanations of/for why...

However, contrary to our hypothesis...

5. 指出局限性,提出今后的研究方向

Controversy still exists as to/regarding...

The discrepancies between...and...may be due to...

Further work/study should include...

6. 指出理论意义、实际应用和潜在价值

It was verified/confirmed that...

A surprising finding was that...

The research on...provides an experimental basis for the use of...and expands to the potential value of...

The identification of...should be a starting point to do..., adding a new dimension to the understanding of..., and assisting sb. in doing...

练习

1. 用讨论的规范用语改写下列句子。

（1）In contrast to these results, Packer et al considered that the RNA level of MUC13 was decreased in colon cancer.

（2）Our data showed that we obtained miRNA expression profiles of BCSCs, which provided a substantial basis for exploring the function of miRNAs in maintaining stem cell properties and the biological functions of BCSCs.

（3）Besides, we also detected the expression of some predicted miRNAs in the BCSCs.

（4）Excitedly, several AITD（autoimmune thyroid disease）susceptibility genes have been identified and characterized.

（5）To confirm that *DNMT3A* repressing the expression of *Oct4* is through altering the degree of DNA methylation, we analyzed the DNA methylation status in three key regions of *Oct4* by BGS.

（6）Rapid detection is the most prominent advantage of this method; the sample detection step can be finished within 15 min.

2. 翻译下列句子。

（1）_____（我们报道了……的新方法）of isolating decision-making circuits and for relating broad scale circuit structure to the dynamic behavior of single cells.

（2）_____ The steady-state levels of progerin in LmnanHG/+MEFs and tissues were lower,（对……提出一种可能的解释）the milder phenotypes.

（3）_____（对于……仍存在争议）the use of washed versus unwashed salvaged blood, as discussed.

（4）_____（我们的研究结果支持这种假说）of an underlying autoimmune pathomechanism underlying this rare disease.

（5）However, _____（与我们的假设相反）, propranolol-treated subjects were

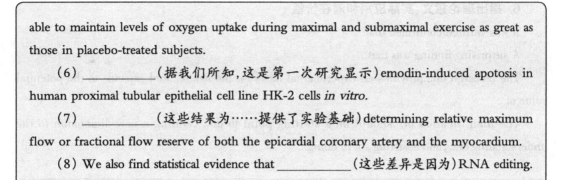

able to maintain levels of oxygen uptake during maximal and submaximal exercise as great as those in placebo-treated subjects.

(6) _____（据我们所知，这是第一次研究显示）emodin-induced apotosis in human proximal tubular epithelial cell line HK-2 cells *in vitro*.

(7) _____（这些结果为……提供了实验基础）determining relative maximum flow or fractional flow reserve of both the epicardial coronary artery and the myocardium.

(8) We also find statistical evidence that _____（这些差异是因为）RNA editing.

（周茜）

第九节 结 论

结论（conclusion）作为一篇论文的结束部分，是整个课题研究的归结所在。结论应该鲜明准确、简短有力，总结说明本研究结果有什么新发现、提出或完善了什么理论、适用于什么样的范围、有什么创新之处或局限性。因此，结论是作者通过前期研究得出的最后见解，是整篇论文的归宿。结论部分应根据研究实验结果，围绕引言提出的研究目的，运用归纳、分析、推理、比较等方法，探讨涉及的问题，说明本研究的理论和实践意义，实事求是地评价研究工作的缺陷，说明有待解决的问题，并提出今后的研究方向。

一、结论的内容

结论部分一般可以分为三个模块，即：

（一）总结模块

回顾前文，概述论文研究内容。在此模块中，一般用一两句话简洁概括即可。

例 1 **In the present work, the results of** experimental, analytical and numerical study into the buckling behaviors of spherical shells **are presented, as well as the effects** of constitutive modes on the buckling loads of these shells.

例 2 **In the present study, we demonstrate** that VEGFR2-induced up-regulation of EC markers is mediated by the activation of ERK signaling pathway, whereas p38 and JNK had no effect on this process. The activation of ERK pathway resulted in a negative crosstalk with JNK pathway, and inhibited JNK phosphorylation. Hence, further *in vivo* studies would support the findings.

本模块中常用句型如下：

The observation results are consistent/in accord with the theory/idea/proposal/hypothesis/previous studies/that...

The experiments/results/findings/investigation/facts supply a basis for...

The results demonstrate/confirm/suggest/indicate/reveal/highlight/cover that...

We have reported the results from...

We have presented the systematic results of...

The study shows that...

We conclude that/Our conclusion is that/It is our conclusion that...

（二）结论模块

提炼结果与讨论中得出的重要论点，指出本论文的创新点和潜在应用价值。

例 3 This work therefore **indicates that** the real load-carrying capacity of a spherical shell can be obtained numerically from measured geometric shape and average wall thickness, as well as from the assumption of elastic-perfectly plastic material properties. **The current approach appears to be effective** for other shells of revolution with typical meridional profiles, such as cylindrical and conical shells, as well as for shells of revolution with nontypical meridional profiles, such as barreled and egg-shaped shells.

例 4 ATR2 silencing showed no effect on AMSC differentiation to ECs. These findings **provide new insights into** the role of VEGFR2 and the ERK signaling pathway in AMSC differentiation to ECs for the potential clinical uses of AMSCs. A large number of clinical trials with long-term follow-up would enhance our understanding of the therapeutic efficiency of AMSCs in regenerative medicine.

本模块中常用句型如下：

A major new finding of this study is that...

To the best of our knowledge, this is the first time that...

A new approach is presented to analyze...

It is also surprising to see virtually...

This is the first study into...

Our study opens avenues for...

Considering that..., this methodology could be a good guideline for...

（三）方向模块

总结方法、结果与讨论中存在的问题，展望下一步研究方向。

例 5 **However, some limitations merit attention.** Although the predicted buckling loads and final failure modes were verified experimentally, the critical buckling modes were not examined through testing. Moreover, the manufacturing process caused some variance in the wall thickness, and that variance exerted an effect on the buckling of spherical shells; however, this effect was not studied. **These limitations require further investigation in the near future.**

例 6 Famitinib did show substantial anti-tumor activities with a good safety profile in heavily pretreated patients with HER2-negative breast cancer. Famitinib-related TSH increase may be an early indicator of its efficacy. Serial monitoring of serum TSH may help define VEGFR2-dependent or VEGFR2-independent drug resistance. **This patient-related rather than tumor-related factor**

should be further assessed in future trials.

本模块中常用句型如下：

Whether...remains/is yet to be determined.

Further analysis/experiments will be necessary/needed to confirm...

The new concept shall be expanded to...

The effect of...has not been examined.

The influence of...was not part of this investigation.

One specific drawback seems to be associated with...

We think/believe/vision/propose/hypothesize/recommend that...

二、结论的写作要求

1. 准确总结，客观严谨　精炼地概括论文中创新的内容。

2. 具体明确，言简意赅　结论应提供明确、具体的定性与定量的信息。对要点要具体表述，不能用抽象和笼统的语言。

3. 综合分析，客观评估　浓缩表达，言之有据。

三、结论写作的人称和时态

（一）人称

结论中不使用 I、my 等代词，而较多地使用 we、our 等代词，从而说明该工作是由多人合作完成；句子主语多为复数形式，以说明结果是在对较广泛的数据进行研究后得出的，具有客观性和广泛性。

例 7　In closing, **our findings** show that **adult SCs** in the HF become active and self-renew by mechanisms that appear to involve mostly non-PcG regulated genes and a bimodal switch involving PcG-regulation is critical to control fate determination and lineage progression. In normal homeostasis, this rheostat does not trigger until multiple signaling inputs converge on the activated HF-SCs, unveiling a requirement for both transcriptional effectors and histone modifications in governing the complex processes of tissue homeostasis and regeneration.

（二）时态

结论部分的时态比较复杂，应注意以下几点：

1. 普遍适用的结论，可用一般现在时。

例 8　Cholesterol efflux capacity from macrophages, a metric of HDL function, **has** a strong inverse association with both carotid intima-media thickness and the likelihood of angiographic coronary disease, independency of the HDL cholesterol level.

巨噬细胞的胆固醇流出量（一种高密度脂蛋白功能的度量指标），与颈动脉内膜中层厚度和经血管造影确诊冠状动脉疾病的可能性均具有强负相关性，其独立于高密度脂蛋白胆固醇水平。

2. 描述本文研究结果且该结论为研究结束时的结论,则用一般过去时。

例 9 In this large European study, a modest increase in protein content and a modest reduction in the glycemic index **led** to an improvement in study completion and maintenance of weight loss.

在这项大规模欧洲研究中,适度增加蛋白量和适度降低血糖指数更有利于研究的完成和降低体重的持续性。

3. 阐述对本研究的预期效果或展望,可用一般现在时或将来时,也可用情态动词形式。表达客观、委婉的看法或建议时,可用 should do 的句子结构表达。

例 10 In outpatients suspected of venous thromboembolism, point of care D-dimer tests **can** contribute important information and guide patient management, notably in low-risk patients (that is, those patients with a low score on a clinical decision rule).

在可疑静脉血栓栓塞的门诊患者中,床旁 D-二聚体检测能够提供重要信息并指导治疗,在低风险患者(即临床决策规则评分较低的患者)中的价值尤为显著。

练习

1. 把下列汉语句子翻译成英语。

(1) 检测 VEGF(血管内皮生长因子)表达可作为胃癌的预后指标,有助于为术后患者的放疗、化疗的选择提供依据。

(2) 下调受刺激内皮细胞 TF 表达的同时上调 TM 表达可能是 GAG 发挥抗血栓形成作用的主要机制之一。

(3) 这些结果与在妊娠妇女中使用丁丙诺啡作为阿片样物质依赖的一种可接受的治疗方法相一致。

2. 把下列英语段落翻译成汉语。

(1) The physiologic changes of pregnancy can reveal risk of chronic diseases. Exaggerated responses reflective of the metabolic syndrome are seen in preeclampsia and gestational diabetes and can herald future cardiovascular and metabolic disease. Pregnancy is therefore an important screening opportunity for cardiovascular and metabolic disease risk factors, with the possibility of early intervention.

(2) In conclusion, the present study demonstrated that the compound Chinese medicine CG is able to attenuate I/R-induced brain edema by interference in tight junction protein degradation and caveolin-1 expression in vascular endothelial cells, accompanying by an improvement in cerebral infarction and neurological score, suggesting CG as a promising alternative approach for the patients at risk to develop severe brain edema.

(周茜)

第十节　参 考 文 献

参考文献(reference)是指为撰写论文或编写论著而引用的图书期刊资料。在学术论文的撰写过程中,经常需要直接或间接地引用其他学者的理论或观点,或者参考相关的文献或著作。

参考文献的格式没有统一的标准,不同的学术研究机构、出版社、杂志社等都有单独制定的要求,供作者参考。原则上,不属于自己原创的内容,都要列出出处,并给出完整文献名称。之所以这样做,一是对原作者的肯定和尊重,避免抄袭和剽窃的嫌疑,二是能为自己的研究提供充分的论据,突出独立创新内容。因此,大部分学术论文审稿专家都十分重视参考文献,甚至将其作为最先审查的内容。

一、引用参考文献的原则和要求

1. 精选最新、最主要的文献资料。如果可能,引用最新的、公开发表和出版的文献资料,以便于读者查阅和核对。引用的论文应为代表相关课题研究水平现状且在权威或专业性杂志上发表的高质量文章,以表现作者对研究内容的熟悉程度,突显本研究的深度和广度。

2. 尽可能引用原始文献。所引文献必须由作者亲自阅读和查阅,确保文献标注的准确性。不可照搬、照抄他人论文中引用的内容,以免出现引用和标注错误。

3. 文献引用要符合投稿要求。不同期刊对参考文献的格式有着不同的要求,甚至对文献的数量也有规定和限制,因此,投稿之前务必认真阅读投稿指南,注意格式上的相关细节,避免返工。

二、参考文献的格式

英文学术论文参考文献的引用和编排规则中最常用的格式有温哥华格式、APA、MLA 等三种格式。它们在文中的引用形式、内容、标点符号、编排顺序上都有一定的区别,需要仔细辨别。

(一) 温哥华格式

温哥华格式(Vancouver style),也称温哥华注释体系(Vancouver system)。该格式要求在正文中所引用的段落后标记数字序号,用来索引文后参考文献,因此也被称为作者-序号体系(author-number system)。

温哥华格式在生物医学和物理科学中比较流行,医学界知名数据库 Medline 和 PubMed 即采用这一格式。1978 年,由各大医学期刊的编辑组成的国际医学期刊编辑委员会(International Committee of Medical Journal Editors,ICMJE)在加拿大温哥华举办会议,制定了《生物医学期刊的原稿统一要求》(Uniform Requirements for Manuscripts Submitted to Biomedical Journals),选定了"作者-序号"体系作为统一的参考文献格式要求,经多次修订后形成了目前国际生物医学界通用的温哥华格式。

温哥华格式规定,参考文献清单按照文中所引文献出现的顺序编排,并使用阿拉伯数字进行编号。因此,正文中引用文献时,出现引用的文段应使用数字对文献依次编号,其形式为括号 + 阿拉伯数字,如(1)、[1]、上标的 1 或者上标加方括号的[1]。数字往往紧跟在参考文字后,或者正文中出现过的参考信息的一部分(如作者姓名、出版年份等)后。例如:

Hypovolemia is a massive decrease in blood volume, and death by excessive loss of blood is referred to as exsanguination.[1] Typically, a healthy person can endure a loss of 10%–15% of the total blood volume without serious medical difficulties.

如上所示,在正文后参考文献清单中的第 1 项即可找到文中所引文献的相关资料。

温哥华格式中关于参考文献格式和编排规则的规定是根据美国国立医学图书馆《医学索引》中的格式确定的。一般情况下,文献作者姓氏为全称,名为缩写形式,且通常省略缩写点;作者为六人以内时全部列出,超过六人时则只列前三名,后加 *et al.* 表明省略;期刊名称如需使用缩写,应统一参照《医学索引》中的标准缩写格式;文摘、未公开发表的观察报告及个人通信不能作为参考文献。下面具体介绍温哥华格式的参考文献编排规则。

著作:作者姓名(先姓后名,如果为两位或两位以上作者,则使用逗号——隔开,下同),著作名称(斜体,需大写所有实词的首字母),出版地,出版单位(与出版地使用冒号隔开,后使用分号),出版年份(后使用句点)。例如:

Eisen HN. *Immunology: An Introduction to Molecular and Cellular Principles of the Immune Response. 5th ed.* New York: Harper and Row; 1974.

Simons NE, Menzies B, Mathews M. *A Short Course in Soil and Rock Slop Engineering.* London: Thomas Telford Publishing; 2001.

Rang HP, Dale MM, Ritter JM, Moore PK, *et al. Pharmacology.* Edinburgh: Churchill Livingstone; 2003.

书中章节:作者姓名,章节名称,编辑姓名(格式同作者,前面使用 In 引出,后使用括号注明 eds.),著作名称(斜体,大写首词的首字母),出版地,出版单位(与出版地使用冒号隔开,后使用分号),出版年份,页码(与出版年份之间使用冒号隔开,后使用句点)。例如:

Weinstein L, Swartz MN. Pathogenic properties engineering of invading microorganisms. In: Sodeman MA Jr, Sodeman WA (eds.) *Pathologic physiology: mechanisms of disease.* Philadelphia: WB Saunders; 1974: 457-72.

Moran MJ. Thermodynamics. In: Kreith F, Goswami DY (eds.) *The CRC handbook of mechanical engineering.* BocaRaton: CRC Press; 2005: 75-81.

期刊文章:作者姓名,文章标题(需大写首词的首字母,不使用斜体),期刊名称(斜体,大写所有实词的首字母或使用标准缩写形式),出版年份(与期刊名称之间不使用标点,后使用分号),卷号,页码(与卷号之间使用冒号隔开,后加句点)。例如:

Ettlin DA. Pemphigus. *Dent Clin North Am* 2005; 49: 107-25.

You Ch, Lee KP, Chey RY, Menguy R. Electrogastrograpic study of patients with unexplained nausea, bloating and vomting. *Gastroenterology* 1980; 79: 311-4.

Shamim T, Varghese VI, Shameena PM, *et al.* Pemphigus vulgaris in oral cavity: clinical analysis of 71 cases. *Med Oral Patol Oral Cir Bucal* 2008;13:E622-6.

如果作者为某研究团队,则用团队名称替代作者姓名;如果作者不详,则用 anonymous (后加句点)替代作者姓名,或者直接以文章标题起始,其余内容格式不变。例如:

The Royal Marsden Hospital Bone-Marrow Transplantation Team. Failure of syngeneic bone-marrow graft without preconditioning in post-hepatitis marrow aplasia. *Lancet* 1997;2:242-4.

Coffee drinking and cancer of the pancreas. Br Med J 2010;283:628.

学位论文:作者姓名,文章标题,学位论文类型,单位,年份。例如:

Leckenby RJ. Dynamic characterization and fluid flow modeling of fractured reservoirs. PhD thesis, Imperial College London;2005.

公开出版的会议论文:作者姓名,文章标题,编辑姓名,会议名称(或论文集名称,使用斜体,大写首词的首字母),出版地,出版单位,出版年份(标点格式同著作)。

DuPont B. Bone Marrwo transplantation in severe combined immunodeficiency with an unrelated MlC compatible donor. In:White HJ, Smith R, eds. *Proceedings of the third annual meeting of the International Society for Experimental Hematology.* New York:Raven Press;1995.

报纸文章:作者姓名,文章标题,报纸名称(斜体,大写所有实词首字母),出版日期(顺序为星期、月、日、年,其间不使用标点符号,星期可省略),页码(与日期间使用冒号隔开)。例如:

Shaffer RA. Advances in chemistry are starting to unlock mysteries of the brain:discoveries could help cure alcoholism and insomnia, explain mental illness. *Wall Street Journal.* Friday Aug 12 1977:12.

Macalister T. Green energy is the modern gold rush. *The Guardian.* Wednesday Jul 2 2008:27.

如果为网络报纸文章,则需标明网址及检索时间。例如:

Pagnamenta R. Energy adviser puts forwards powerful case for hydrogen. *The Times.* May 24 2008. http://business. timesoline. co. uk/tol/business/industry_ sectors/natural_ resources/article 3994594. ece(accessed 2 July 2008).

(二) APA 格式

APA 是美国心理学会(American Psychological Association)所制定的一种参考文献格式,主要用于心理学、教育学、社会科学等学科的论文写作中。APA 格式使用哈佛大学文章引用格式,通常来说,一个引用包含了作者姓氏和发表日期,中间以逗号隔开,以括号加注,格式为(作者姓氏,日期),放在引用文字或句子之后,文献的详细信息则放在位于文章最后的参考文献清单(Reference)部分。

APA 格式规定文献清单部分中的人名必须以姓(family name)的字母顺序来排列。因此,清单中所有类型的文献作者姓名均以姓氏开头,名可以使用首字母缩写,例如,James Smith 应缩写成 Smith, J.,Saif Al Falasi 应缩写成 Al-Falasi, Saif。文献前不使用数字序号,也不用标明文献类型。但是,不同文献类型的格式有所不同,下面予以具体说明。

著作:作者姓名(先姓后名,中间以逗号隔开,如果为两位或两位以上作者,则使用逗号隔开,最后一位与前一位之间使用 & 连接),出版年份(放于括号内,后用句号),著作名称(斜

体,名称中只需大写第一个词的首字母),出版地,出版单位。例如:

Watkins, P. J. (2003). *ABC of diabetes. 5thed.* London:Blackwell Publishing.

Smith, J., & Peter, Q. (1992). *Hairball:An intensive peek behind the surface of an Enigma.* Hamilton:McMaster University Press.

Simons, N. E., Menzies, B., & Mathews, M. (2001). *A short course in soil and rock slop engineering.* London:Thomas Telford Publishing.

注意,如果作者人数超过六人,则不必全部列出,只需在列举出前六位之后使用 *et al.* 即可。

文集中的文章:作者姓名(用法同著作),出版年份,著作名称,文章标题(斜体,只需大写句首字母),页码(放于括号中),出版地,出版单位。例如:

McDonalds, A. (1993). Practical methods for the apprehension and sustained containment of supernatural entities. *Paranormal and occult studies:case studies in application* (pp. 42–64). London:Other World Books.

期刊与报纸文章:作者姓名,出版年份,文章标题(斜体,只需大写句首字母,后使用句号),期刊名称,期/卷/号,页码。例如:

Herbst, A., &Bystryn, J. C. (2000). *Patterns of emission in pemphigus.* Canadian/American Studies Journal, 42, 2-7.

Rosenbach, M., Murrell, D. F., Bystryn, J. C., *et al.* (2009). *Reliability and convergent validity of two outcome instruments for pemphigus.* J Invest Dermmatol, 129, 4-10.

学位论文:作者姓名,完成时间,论文标题(用法同期刊与报纸文章),层次及是否公开发表,单位(学校、研究所等),单位所在地。例如:

Huan, C. P. (2015). *Journalist stance in Chinese and Australian hard news.* Unpublished doctorial dissertation, Macquarie University, Sydney.

网络期刊的文章:作者姓名,出版年份,文章标题(斜体),期刊名称,期号,文章编号,检索日期,网站(使用 from 引出)。注意,结尾不使用任何标点符号。例如:

Blofeld, E. S. (1994, March 1). *Expressing oneself through Persian cats and modern architecture.* Felines & Felons, 4, Article 0046g. Retrieved October 3, 1999, from http://jbr. org./ article. html

(三) MLA 格式

MLA (Modern Language Association)是一种人文领域常用的引用格式,为美国现代语言协会制定的论文指导格式,常用于文学、艺术等学科,强调文献引用的完整性。MLA 格式规定,文中引用格式为"(作者姓氏页码)",姓氏与页码之间空格即可,不使用标点符号,也不用标注年份。其参考文献编排格式与 APA 也有一定区别,下文将具体说明。

MLA 格式中参考文献清单写作 Bibliography 或者 Works Cited,文献按照作者姓氏的首字母顺序排列。如果作者不详,则使用文献名称的首字母进行排序,但是文献名称中的 a, an, the 三个词不参与排序。与 APA 格式类似,各文献前不使用数字序号,也不用标明文献类型。常用文献类型格式如下:

著作：作者姓名（先姓后名，中间以逗号隔开），著作名称（斜体，名称中所有实词的首字母均须大写，后使用句号），出版地，出版单位（出版地与出版单位之间用冒号连接），出版年份。例如：

Myant, N. B. *The Biology of Cholesterol and Related Steroid.* London：Heinemann Medical Books, 1981.

如果著作为两人共同完成，格式为：第一作者姓名（先姓后名，使用逗号隔开），第二作者姓名（正常顺序，与第一作者姓名用 and 连接，如果为缩写名，则仍保持先姓后名的格式），著作名称（斜体），出版地，出版单位（出版地与出版单位之间用冒号连接），出版年份。三人或三人以上共同完成的著作可以在第一作者姓名后面使用 *et al.* 表示省略。例如：

Horton, Rod W., and Herbert W. Edwards. *Backgrounds of American Literary Thought*. New York：Appleton-Century-Crofts, Inc., 1952.

Belenky, Mary Field, *et al. Women's Ways of Knowing：The Development of Self, Voice and Mind*. New York：Basic, 1986.

学术期刊文章：作者姓，名，文章标题（使用引号），期刊名称（斜体，与期号之间不使用标点），期号，出版年（使用括号标出），页码范围（与出版年之间使用冒号连接）。两位或两位以上作者的列出格式参考以上著作的格式。例如：

独立作者：

Steinberg, A. D. "Cyclonphospamide：Should It Be Used Daily, Monthly, or Never?". *N Engl J Med* 310（1984）：458-459.

两位作者：

Zhao, C. Y. and Murrell, D. F. "Pemphigus Vulgaris：an Evidence-based Treatment". *Drugs* 75（2015）：271-284.

三位或三位以上作者：

Mascia-Lees, F.E., Sharpe, P., and Cohen, C.B. . "Double Liminality and the Black Woman Writer". *American Behavioral Scientist* 31（1987）：101-104.

或者，

Mascia-Lees, F.E., *et al*. "Double Liminality and the Black Woman Writer". *American Behavioral Scientist* 31（1987）：101-104.

普通杂志与报纸文章：格式与学术杂志文章类似，需另外标明报纸或杂志出版的具体日期和版面（版面与出版日期之间使用冒号）。例如：

Di Rado, Alicia. "Trekking through College：Classes Explore Modern Society Using the World of Star Trek". *Los Angeles Times* 15 Mar. 1995：A3.

网络期刊文章：格式与学术杂志文章类似，需在最后标出检索地点和时间。例如：

Lynch, Tim. "DSN Trials and Tribble-ations Review". *Psi Phi：Bradley's Science Fiction Club.* 1996. Bradley University. 8 Oct. 1997.

Andreadis, Athena. "The Enterprise Finds Twin Earths Everywhere It Goes, But Future

Colonizers of Distant Planets Won't Be So Lucky". *Astronomy* Jan. 1999：64. Lexis-Nexis Academic Universe. B. Davis Schwartz Memorial Library，Brookville，NY. 7 Feb. 1999.

本节内容简要介绍了英文学术论文参考文献部分的写作目的、原则和三种常用参考文献格式，相关格式在官方网站上有更为详细的要求和规则。即便要求采用某一通用格式，各期刊在具体细节上也可能存在细微差别。因此，作者在投稿之前务必仔细阅读目标期刊的投稿指南（Guide for Authors），按照其中的具体格式要求和示例撰写参考文献部分，以便文章顺利通过审核。目前，文献导入时也可以使用 endnote、NoteExpress、mendeley 等文献管理软件进行，导入完成后再予以核对和手动修正，较为方便快捷，可根据需要选择相关软件学习使用。

练习

以下内容摘自某医学专业论文的文献清单，请尝试以温哥华格式进行编排。

Blasi，F.（2004）*Atypical Pathogens and Respiratory Tract Infections.* European Respiratory Journal，55，23-25.

Burillo，A.，Bouza，E.（2010）*Chlamydophila Pneumoniae Infect.* Dis Clin North Am，10，72-74.

Ciarrocchi，G.，Benedetto，F.，Fogliani，V.，*et al.*（2004）*Serological Study on Chlamydophila Pneumoniae in Patients with Community-acquired Pneumonia.* Garcia-Jardon，M.，Bhat V. G.，Blanco-Blanco，E.，*et al.*（2010）*Postmortem Findings in HIV/AIDS Patients in a Tertiary Care Hospital in Rural South Africa.* Tropical Doctor，2，11-13.

Kuo，C. C. & Campbell，L. A.（2003）*Chlamydial Infections of the Cardiovascular System.* Frontiers in Bioscience，12，34-38.

Lee，S. J.，Lee，M. G.，Jeon，M. J.，*et al.*（2002）*Atypical Pathogens in Adult Patients Admitted with Community-acquired Pneumonia in Korea.* Japanese Journal of Infectious Diseases，8，112-114.

Miyashita，N.，Obase，Y.，Fukuda，M.，*et al.*（2006）*Evaluation of Serological Tests Detecting Chlamydophila Pneumoniae-specific Immunoglobulin M Antibody.* Journal of Internal Medicine，23，112-115.

Miyashita，N.，Kawai，Y.，Yamaguchi，T.，*et al.*（2010）*Evaluation of False Positive Reaction with ELISA for the Detection of Chlamydophila Pneumoniae-specific IgM Antibody in Adults.* Japanese Journal of Infectious Diseases，32，76-78.

Satpalhy，G.，Sharma，A. & Vasisht，S.（2005）*Immunocomb Chlamydia Bivalent Assay to Study Chlamydia Species Specific Antibodies in Patients with Coronary Heart Disease.* Indian Journal of Medical Research，7，53-55.

（韩涛）

第三章 留学文书写作

近年来,越来越多的本科毕业生及研究生计划在结束本阶段的学习和研究之后前往国外的高校或研究机构深造。申请者除了必须具备一定的学业成绩、学术成就、语言能力等之外,还需要准备一套完整的留学申请材料。其中,留学文书的准备和写作可以最大限度地展示申请人的个性、才智、学术观点和成就,以及研究计划、目标和潜力等,有助于增加申请人的录取机会。

留学文书主要包括个人陈述(Personal Statement)、个人简历(Resume)和推荐信(Recommendation Letter)等。

第一节 个 人 陈 述

个人陈述(Personal Statement),也称为 admissions essay,是所有留学文书中最为重要的一部分。其写作目的是充分反映申请人的个性特点和才智,全面展示申请人的学术观点、学术成就、研究潜力、领导能力、组织协调能力以及其他方面的特殊才能。因此,从某种意义上讲,一份主题鲜明、内容充实的个人陈述对于能否申请成功具有决定性作用。

一、写作准备

个人陈述的写作绝不是一蹴而就的,需要进行充分的准备,设计合理的结构。准备工作包括进行个人评估、做好调查研究、考虑招生委员会提出的问题等。

1. **个人评估** 个人评估是申请人对自己的各方面予以全面客观的评价。这项工作需要花费一定的时间和精力,推荐采用写作中常见的头脑风暴法(brainstorming)。首先,准备纸质或电子的书写材料,开始记录下脑海中出现的所有内容,重点描述愿望、梦想、抱负等。例如,自己希望从研究生阶段的学习和研究中获得什么?

当然,此类信息并非必须全部包含在个人陈述中。此时的目标是将所有内容一一列出,以供下一步选取使用。因此,尽可能将自己的个人经历逐条列出,以便后期筛选出对个人陈述有意义和增强作用的内容。可以着重记录以下几个方面的内容:①兴趣爱好;②已完成的研究项目或在学术领域的成就;③为自身带来巨大变化的人生经历;④参与过的挑战和克服过的困难;⑤激发受教育积极性的相关经历;⑥具有重要影响作用的关键人物;⑦对成功具有决定性作用的个性、品质、工作习惯、态度等。

结合自己的学业成绩和学术成就,努力找出其与上面所列内容之间的联系,并一一对应起来。例如,好奇心与求知欲引领自己在教授的指导下完成了某项独立研究。

揣摩每项对应内容是否能够表明自己已经为未来的研究和学习做好充分的准备。此外,还需考虑如何将这些内容运用到个人陈述的写作之中。

确定一份总清单之后,认真检查清单中所列出的内容和信息。需要注意的是,最终在个人陈述中使用的内容应当有助于将申请人刻画为一个积极乐观的人,而非一个疲惫沮丧的学生。据此进一步修改主清单,审慎决定是否将某项内容纳入个人陈述之中。修改完成后,即可将这份清单作为后面撰写个人陈述的基础内容。

2. 调查研究　调查研究吸引自己申请留学的项目。认真阅读宣传材料,浏览网页内容,多渠道搜集一切能够帮助了解招生委员会对未来学生要求和希望的信息。这样做可以为接下来的个人陈述写作提供所申请学校或机构充足的相关知识,以展示自己对学校或研究机构的兴趣以及对研究项目所做的功课。要着重记录与前文总结的个人特质、兴趣、已取得的成就等内容一致或相关的内容。

3. 思考招生委员会提出的问题　多数招生委员会要求申请人在个人陈述中回答一系列的具体问题。例如:Please tell us your reasons for applying for graduate study, your particular area of specialization within your field of study./What is the biggest challenge you have faced and how will you overcome it? 尽管许多问题都是老生常谈,写作时还是应该注意是否做出了回答,回答的内容是否符合文章主旨,是否与头脑风暴中列出的总清单条目相一致。注意回答应尽可能简洁明了,避免冗长繁杂。

写作前,应熟悉个人陈述的基本结构。写作过程中应始终牢记,这是展示自己的能力与闪光点的绝好机会,务必充分利用。此外,招生委员会一般由专业人员组成,他们已经阅读过成百上千甚至更多申请者的个人陈述。因此,一定要设法使自己的文章与众不同,才能脱颖而出。

总之,撰写个人陈述就如同为招生委员会讲一个故事,一个关于自己是谁以及能做些什么的故事。尽管不同的学校和研究项目提出的问题不尽相同,但是重点和难点都是如何去推荐自己,呈现一个成功候选人的潜力。

二、文章结构与内容组织

个人陈述有几种不同的结构形式,最常用的包含简介、正文和结语三个部分。

1. 简介　简介是个人陈述的开篇,是对整篇文章的介绍和导入。简介应设法吸引读者的兴趣,愿意继续读下去。因此,开篇一定要独特且引人注目,尽可能使其发人深省或引起关注。简介可以阐述申请人对某个专业课题研究的强烈愿望,或者探讨引发申请人对某个课题的兴趣并希望进行研究的动机。尽可能采用较有创意的方式陈述和讨论这些内容。下面几篇样文可供参考。

例 1　From an early age, I have been fascinated by the workings of life. The human body is a remarkable machine with many diverse systems producing an organism that could never be artificially reproduced. My love of science is just one of my reasons for choosing medicine. I enjoy a challenge particularly towards an objective and although medicine is a tough career it can be enormously gratifying, highlighted by the doctors I have spoken to during my experience and on a personal level.

短短几句话包含了丰富的信息,包括学医的决心、从医经验以及对医学专业的理解等,简洁明了且均为有效信息。

例 2 The great businessman Lee Iacocca is accredited with saying, "You've got to say that I think that if I keep working at this and want it badly enough I can have it. It's called perseverance." This quote struck a chord with me, especially as I set out to attain my own professional desires and academic goals via entering MSc Management Science at the London School of Economics and Political Science. I am eager to appeal to you as to why my past experience and future professional intent make me a nature fit for this prestigious program.

申请人开篇引用名人名言,与专业巧妙联系起来。思路清晰,引出下文内容,从 past experience 和 future professional intent 两方面论述为什么他是所申请专业最合适的人选。

此外,申请人还可以通过描述特殊事例引出专业选择的具体原因。

例 3 As I was finishing college, my mother had both her hips replaced with artificial ones because all of the cartilage in her hip joints had worn away and it was very painful for her to walk. I found it fascinating that engineers, orthopedic surgeons and biologists had all worked together to design these artificial joints that completely transform people's lives by giving them back pain-free mobility, and I knew at that moment that this was an area about which I wanted to learn more.

申请人以母亲的手术经历作为开篇,成功引出自己对整形医学产生兴趣的由来,解释专业选择的具体原因。

2. 正文 正文是文章的主体部分,一般包含三个或更多段落,为简介提供细节证明和支撑。段落之间需要进行必要的过渡,做到衔接连贯、行文流畅。

各个段落应着重探讨以下几个方面的内容:专业兴趣、以往的学习经历和表现、社会实践经历、学校选择及职业规划等。专业兴趣可以从家庭影响、兴趣起源等方面说明,提供具体事例,说明个人在成长过程中积累专业知识的能力。

例 4 After four years' efforts, including thorough theory studies and ample research work, traditional Chinese medicine, once an entirely unfamiliar concept to me, has now become my career objective.

申请研究生学习时,本科阶段的专业更容易让招生委员会看到学生的潜力。如果所申请专业与原来所学专业无关,需要详细说明改变专业的动机、目的、过程等。

例 5 Studies in my undergraduate major, psychology, require practical experience, from which I become aware of the spirit of psychology and confirm my determination of further pursue in this field. Out of many experiences, the time when I served as a volunteer in the year-long project of Growth Guide (aiming to serve children who have experienced Sichuan earthquake) most inspired this decision.

对于过去的学习经历和表现,申请人可以按照时间顺序介绍(例 6),也可以具体描述课堂表现,例如理解能力、反应能力、接受新知识的能力等,其中也可加入获得过优异成绩的演讲、参与完成的项目、实验经历等。语言应该避免平铺直叙，可以强调学习过程中遇到的困难、解决的过程等，以突出个人解决问题的能力、抗压能力及潜力。此外，也可以简单介绍曾经参加过的学术活动、学生社团活动等，说明自己的竞争能力、领导能力、组织协调能力及团队协作能力等（例7）。

例6 The first two years of my academic studies were focused on sharpening my basic skills of listening, writing, reading, and speaking in English. They provided me with confidence in my command of English. Starting in my junior years, we delved into the different branches of our major, Literature, Linguistics and English Education. I enjoyed all the courses from different aspects, but what interested me most was linguistics, especially theories related to second language acquisition.

例7 My research capacity, creative thinking and experimental skills experienced further improvement as I joined a research group at the XX Research Institute of Digestive Diseases to undertake a research project for my Master's program. Under the leadership of Prof. Jin, the most celebrated specialist on digestion, I participated in the project The Development of Chronic Stomach Disease (Gastrosia) & The Mechanism of Concretization sponsored by Hebei Provincial Bureau of Public Health. In this project, I focused my research on the mechanism of action and the cellular immunity of the catalyst subunit telomerase in cancerization and investigated, through a microscopic approach, the clinical significance that those two factors may produce on the diagnosis, treatment and prognosis of the gastric cancer.

社会实践主要指申请人曾经参加过的志愿者服务活动、实习、工作、接受培训等经历，以表现实践能力和工作潜力。应写明实践的单位、时间、地点、工作过程、担任的职位及职责、取得的成绩及受到的评价等。

例8 I have accumulated much practical clinical experience since I started working at The No. 2 Hospital of XX Medical University which is classified as the "Grade-A Class-III" hospital (the highest ranking for a hospital in China). Based on my research during the Master's program, I expanded my research area to include the study on gastric cancer. I have published a total of six papers (please refer to my Resume for more detailed information), including the latest The Expression and the Clinical Implication of the Catalyst Subunit Telomerase in Gastric Cancer and Precancerosis, in the *World Journal of Gastroenterology* and other leading journals in China. Some of those papers were designated to be presented at annual conference on digestion in Jiangsu and Guangdong Provinces.

例9 While undertaking research, I have received formal and comprehensive training as resident physician of internal medicine and obtained national doctor license. Through the training program I have grasped the pathogenetic mechanisms of gastrointestinal and liver diseases, cardiovascular diseases, endocrinopathy, pulmonary and connective tissue diseases and their corresponding diagnosis and treatment. In less than two years after working at the hospital, I passed the national-level qualifying examination to have achieved the qualifications as the physician-in-charge in digestive internal medicine.

例 8 首先提到医院的实习经历,进而引出科研方向和论文发表情况,参加培训的经历。例 9 着重介绍项目研究过程中接受的培训,以说明自己通过培训掌握的技能。

关于学校选择,应表明自己独特的见解和观点,尽量避免空话套话,简要介绍自己未来的职业规划,并说明所选学校和专业对个人的未来成长和职业生涯将起到的重要作用。

例 10 Boston College, in my view, can offer me what I want. Firstly, BC aims to teach both professionally and academically. By participating in classes and activities, I surely can enhance my abilities in putting theory into practice and improve my self-reflection ability by guidance. Secondly, I share with BC in its social responsibilities of helping the underprivileged population, which is quite lacking in China. I want to feel this responsibility in the community of BC and strive to do more and do better. Thirdly, Master Program of social work in BC also focuses on diversity. I am convinced that only in such an academic environment can I be exposed to more tolerating academic atmosphere and diverse values and cultivate fertile mind.

正文最后解释说明学校能够录取申请人的原因。

例 11 I have two goals. One is to become a professional social worker both in research and practice. The other is to intervene independently in youth growth, especially the developmental work for youth, intervention for high-risk youth and family guidance. I sincerely believe that systematic study and social experience at Boston College can turn me into a truly qualified social worker.

3. 结语 结语可以总结正文的内容,也可以再次强调开篇内容,表达自己对所申请专业的理解和实现目标的决心。

例 12 I will become a more professional psychiatrist and, with my knowledge and skill, I can help those who are in depression, confusion or other needs, just like what I did years ago, to accompany them walk through the tough period.

三、个人陈述的写作原则

个人陈述的写作应注意遵循以下几个原则:

1. 独特性原则 每个申请人都是独特的,家庭背景、天资禀赋、接受的教育、爱好、经历等都有所不同。所以,在撰写个人陈述时不要盲目模仿他人的文章,要写出自己的独特性,可以是独特的专业素养(例 13),或者是与众不同的性格特征(例 14)。

例 13 Compared with numerous other applicants, I believe that my unique advantage dwells in the strong motivation in life science and in basic medicine that I have maintained over the years. But more importantly, it is embodied by the academic success I have achieved in my 5-year undergraduate education in medical science and in the development of strong ability to perform independent medical research in my 2-year work experience.

例 14 I used to be quite rebellious when I was in junior high school. I felt so wronged that mother could not understand me and insist me doing exactly what she told to. Although my rebellion was suppressed by mother again and again, I would like so much my mother to understand my ideas and solve my problems, rather than mere criticism.

2. 真实性与相关性原则 尽管强调独特性, 申请人在写作时也不应为了与众不同而编造一些哗众取宠的虚假内容。这些内容不但不能成为加分项, 反而可能造成申请失败。此外, 有些申请人会使用很大的篇幅描写一些与申请专业毫不相关的信息, 这样做同样毫无意义。个人陈述篇幅有限, 因而申请人必须在有限的篇幅中设法让招生委员会了解自己选择某个专业的明确目标和强烈动机, 并且具备完成该专业学习和研究的能力和条件。

例 15 As far as I am concerned, I am most interested in the research on auto-immune diseases and on tumor. Specifically, I am very enthusiastic about studying the disequilibrium of the subpopulation of cells in organism caused by those diseases, the role of dendritic cells (DC), and other topics. I would like to approach those issues from such perspectives as the activation of immunocytes, the co-stimulating cells of proliferation, and the activated signal transduction.

例 16 As early as the years when I was an undergraduate at the Department of Medicine of XX (Provincial) Medical University, I had a chance to read the book *The Reach of Helicobacter Pylori* edited by some professors of your university which influenced me to take up the study of digestive diseases as my area of specialization. Later, during my Master's Program, I focused on the development of the chronic stomach disease (gastrosia) and the incidence of the gastric cancer. The comprehensive research and practice that I have performed in this area further reinforce my determination to seek advanced studies at your university when there should be an opportunity.

例 15 直截了当地对个人专业兴趣进行了具体而详尽的说明, 从而展现出申请人在这一领域的知识储备和研究准备; 例 16 则通过求学经历引出对慢性胃病这一研究领域的兴趣是如何逐渐产生和发展的, 表达了强烈的研究决心。

3. 内容具体原则 个人陈述的相关内容应尽可能客观具体, 不要仅仅罗列抽象的评价。比如, 要表现申请人的组织协调能力和解决问题的能力, 不能只用 "I am very good at organizing and coordinating" 或者 "I always do well in resolving problems" 这类语言一语带过, 而应该举出具体的例子进行证明 (例 17), 要突出某方面的特殊技能, 不能只是简单陈述, 同样需要例证进行详细说明 (例 18)。

例 17 I was given the chance to guide some students in Beijing Railway Electrification School and help them organize a team with mutual trust and cooperation. But it is not so easy to be a group leader. A girl, one of my group members, refused to cooperate and feigned indifference. In order to solve this problem, I, together with my team members, did an "original family" in which we shared our ideas about the family member who influenced us most. This proved to be a turning point. She shared with us her family life and what led her to what she was. From then on, I began to get to know her and all group members became more understanding of each other.

例 18 Considering my expertise in database and computer programming design, my advisor assigned me the head of a research group composed of four graduate students and several undergraduate students. I went on three field trips to collect hands-on data, coordinated efforts within the team, sought valuable help from experts at the Department of Computer Science and School of Management in XX University, and actively interacted with people on the development committee of the industrial park. In the end, we successfully completed the project and even exceeded the committee's expectations.

4. 语言规范原则 行文中不能出现语法错误,这是撰写个人陈述的最基本要求。语言简洁流畅,词汇使用适宜,句子长短搭配,力求将所要表达的意思完整清晰地表述出来,不要为了炫耀语言能力而使用罕见的词汇和结构过于复杂的句型,更不能全篇模仿甚至抄袭别人的内容。

5. 重点突出原则 阅读个人陈述时,招生人员希望能看到申请人的主要品质和潜力,例如学术能力、创新能力、团队精神、领导能力等。但是,一个人不可能具备所有的优点和能力。因此,在写作时,尽量突出重点,描述清楚自己最具有优势的几项特质和能力,不要试图面面俱到。

四、个人陈述范文

Personal Statement for Ph. D. in Immunology

To become a successful clinical physician who can be the guardian of human health and life, this was my one-time ambition that I believe I would pursue. However, a memorable experience during my internship prior to the undergraduate graduation completely changed my mind. When I witnessed how a patient suffering from lymphatic cancer was tortured, minute by minute, by the agony of approaching his death and yet had to undergo the immense physical pains brought by chemical therapy, radioactive therapy and other trauma-producing therapeutic measures, I experienced a deep sorrow and regret for my not being able to help him alleviate his pain.

I know that at present clinical level many tough problems still remain unsolved, such as the deciphering of the pathogeny of auto-immune diseases and its corresponding prevention and treatment. Only through colossal research work in immunology will it be possible to arrive at some tentative treatment of such diseases. Therefore, when I graduated from XX Medical College, I decided to stay at my Alma Mater to take up research in immunology, which is closely connected with basic medicine. By now, initial progress has been achieved. Realizing the need to further upgrade my professional knowledge and expertise, I file this application for a Ph. D. program in immunology at the University of XX.

Compared with numerous other applicants, I believe that my unique advantage dwells in the strong motivation in life science and in basic medicine that I have maintained over the years. But more importantly, it is embodied by the academic success I have achieved in my 5-year undergraduate education in medical science and in the development of strong ability to perform independent medical research in my 2-year work experience.

My undergraduate program in clinical medicine encompassed approximately 30 courses across basic medicine and clinical medicine. I was particularly interested in those sub-disciplines of biological science that demand cogent logical analysis and creative thinking. Immunology fascinated me most. That was because it is a science that exploits the principle that the immunological system of all living organisms can produce rejection effect against any alien intruder or against their own mutants and provides completely new solutions to the diverse phenomena displayed by different strains and individual organisms and to their diseases. The concepts and methodologies of immunology promise to solve related problems across different fields. My academic performance during those five years should be described as "outstanding", with my scores ranking first among a total of 280 students in the entire grade. For this, I was awarded special-class Scholarship for Outstanding Student for 6 times throughout my undergraduate career.

Apart from coursework, I participated in academic exchange activities as student representative of our college. In 2000, I made a presentation entitled "A General Description of Cellular Apoptosis and Clinical Application" at the First Youth Forum on Pathology in XX Province and my presentation was given the Winning Prize by professors of pathology present at the forum. In addition to that, I had always made conscious efforts to improve my experimental skills and hands-on abilities. I achieved straight A's in all the internship-related subjects in my last year of undergraduate program, winning the honor of Outstanding Interning Student from the hospital where I interned. In my college itself, I served as the chairman of the Extracurricular Pathological and Pharmacological Study Group, winning first prizes for myself or for my group at various knowledge contests in Human Anatomy, Physiology and Biochemistry, Pathology, and Basic Medicine.

Upon my graduation, I chose to take up a teaching position at my Alma Mater. This gave me the precious opportunity to apply my knowledge and to be further exposed to research. Besides working as a teaching assistant at Microbiology and Immunology Department, I devoted most of my time to advanced self-education in immunology. For two years, I have been responsible for delivering both theoretical and (pre-) experimental courses in microbiology and immunology in the entire college, as well as after-class coaching. I have been the first in my department to propose that educational reform be introduced into our department to adopt the heuristic method of elicitation and bilingual education (Chinese and English). In a project in which my college collaborated with the Medical College of XX University on the preparation of the pool of questions on immunology and microbiology, I was responsible for preparing questions concerning two chapters on immunology and three chapters on microbiology. I audited and self-studied many courses for graduate students and joined in their experiments. I have mastered basic experimental skills in cell biology, molecular biology, immunology and microbiology, ranging from aseptic technique, cell culture, lymphocyte separation, gel electrophoresis, immunoblotting to immunofluorescence technique.

At present, I am undertaking my own research project—Study on the Expression Level of CTLA-4 (Cytotoxic T Lymph Antigen-4) in the CD4+T of Systematic Lupus Erythematosus (SLE).

In view of the relationship between the CTLA-4 as an inhibiting co-stimulating cell and the genesis of SLE and its level of severity, as well as the abnormal pattern of the subpopulation of the T cell in the peripheral blood of the SLE patients, I suggest that, in the genesis and development of the SLE, the abnormal expression of CTLA-4 and other inhibiting cells in T lymph cells can lead to distribution disequilibrium of the subpopulation of T cells in an organism, creating abnormal patterns in immune responses and thereby facilitating the development of this type of auto-immune diseases. The significance of my research project lies in the fact that the pathogeny of the auto-immune diseases in the SLE category can be explicated through the activation of lymph cells and signal transduction in the immunological system. In this way, the view that CTLA-4 is an intervening and regulating point in the prevention of SLE and other auto-immune diseases will receive stronger support and the key to intervention and regulation becomes more likely to be discovered.

As an interdisciplinary subject that is of cutting-edge significance, immunology offers many exciting yet challenging fields for research breakthroughs. As far as I am concerned, I am most interested in the research on auto-immune diseases and on tumor. Specifically, I am very enthusiastic about studying the disequilibrium of the subpopulation of cells in organism caused by those diseases, the role of dendritic cells (DC), and other topics. I would like to approach those issues from such perspectives as the activation of immunocytes, the co-stimulating cells of proliferation, and the activated signal transduction.

To fulfill my aspirations, I deem it necessary to seek a Ph. D. degree from the University of XX. As is universally acknowledged, the United States is performing leading research in basic medicine and your esteemed university enjoys a specially high academic reputation in the field of biomedical research. The famous XX Center is based in your university. The most important factor is that your program offers research fields I am intensely interested in. I believe that your education will broaden my knowledge horizon, expose me to distinguished professors and their original concepts and creative teaching. I will also learn advanced theories of immunology and sophisticated experimental skills.

Ultimately I hope that I can become part of the process that human beings use advanced research findings to decipher the mysteries of life and the genesis of diseases. The early clinical application of those research findings will undoubtedly make our life better.

Signature:

(曲悃)

第二节　个人简历

个人简历(Resume)是对留学申请人的教育背景、工作经历、主要成就和贡献的总结和介绍。招生工作人员通常会根据个人简历的内容判断一位申请人是否符合他们的招生条件,进而确定是否从成千上万名申请者中对其予以录取。因此,在撰写个人简历时,申请人应尽可能突出和强调自身的优势特质。

一、个人简历的写作方法与建议

留学个人简历没有固定格式,不同学校通常会有各自的具体要求,因此在格式上认真参照目标学校的官方网站简历模板即可。下面是个人简历写作过程中需要注意的事情。

1. 言简意赅,直奔主题 个人简历的审阅时间往往不会超过一分钟,因此简历必须结构清晰,重点突出,迅速吸引读者的注意力。一般来讲,简历的长度没有规定,但是,尽可能将其控制在一页之内。如果长达两页或以上,那么很可能第二页之后的内容根本不会被读到。当然,如果涉及的内容较多,则有必要超过一页,因此要灵活掌握。

2. 使用垂直列表和动词短语 同样是由于招生人员阅读个人简历的速度较快,相对于段落而言,垂直列表更为可取。同时,列表中的条目尽可能使用可以形成工整排比句式的动词结构。

例如:介绍个人取得的成绩时可以逐条使用设计(design)、分析(analyze)、组织(organize)、完成(accomplish)等动词,以便进行强调。也可以使用名词性短语,但不要使用以第一人称I开头的陈述句。例如,I assisted in...、I developed the... 等,将主语去掉,直接使用动词过去时即可。

例如,organized school Christmas Party three times,assisted in the chemical nucleic acid enzyme effects of metal complexes studied by Gel Imaging System...

3. 灵活取舍,精选最有必要和最有意义的内容 个人简历中必须包括以下内容:

(1)个人基本信息(Basic Information):简历中首先要呈现申请人的基本信息,包括姓名、性别、出生年月、地址、联系电话、电子邮箱等。其中,邮箱是整个申请中最为重要的沟通工具,如无特殊情况,学校会通过电子邮件与申请者进行必要的联系,而很少会通过拨打电话的形式,即使学校准备进行电话面试,也会事先给申请者发送邮件进行通知和确认。因此,拥有一个申请留学专用邮箱是十分必要的。

例如:

Mr. Zhang Qingbin

Address:P. O. Box1708,Beijing University,Beijing,P. R. China,100875

Email:qingbin118@163. com

Tel:0086-10-6345-7896   Cell phone:0086-15012345678

(2)申请目标(Objective):在简历中说明自己的申请目标会让阅读者感受到尊重,通常只需要一个句子就可以将其说明白,即申请某一年某季节某学位某专业。

例如:Ph. D. in chemistry,April 2018

(3)教育背景(Education Background/Experience):教育背景包括学校教育经历和培训经历。学校教育经历中要说明学校名称、专业、学位名称、成绩排名。注意,如果学校并非国际知名院校,可以在学校名称后以注解形式简单评价就读的学校。是否在简历中列出自己的成绩排名取决于实际排名是否理想,如果排名靠前,则可以作为突出优势列出来,相反,如果排名较差,则可以选择回避。除了学校教育之外,申请者如果还有某些校外培训经历,也可包含在简历中,这些经历同样很有可能成为申请优势之一。例如,临床医学专业的学生参加了校外权威机构组织的康复治疗专业培训并取得证书,显然能够成为个人简历中的亮点。

例如:

Sept. 2011–present:School of Medicine,Beijing University

Major:Medicine

Degree:Master of Medical Science(to be received in June 2019)

Training:Participated in rehabilitation training and attained qualification(2016)

Overall GPA:86.5/100

Major GPA:88.5/100

(4)论文和科研经历(Research Experience and Publications):论文部分不仅包括已经公开发表的文章,还包括一些与专业相关的非学术的文章和正在撰写的论文,因为文章的写作和发表不仅是申请者专业能力的体现,也是其创造力的体现。除了列出文章题目,还可以简要介绍文章内容,着重强调专业相关性和创新性。申请者的科研经历是招生委员会非常看重的内容之一,特别是对于申请研究型学科的申请者而言,研究经历更为重要。介绍研究经历时,着重说明研究过程、研究内容、持续时间、研究结果等。但是,如果没有参与过较大型的研究,可以尝试考虑小型的自主研究,只要涉及统计能力、分析能力、解决问题的能力和研究精神,都属于研究的范畴,不要因为感到自卑而放弃这部分内容。例如:

Research Experience

2015–present:Member of 2015 Beijing University Undergraduate Research Fund Program

Project:The chemical nucleic acid enzyme effects of metal complexes studied by Gel Imaging System

Main job:The synthesis of copper complexes and their effects with plasmid DNA studied by Gel Electrophoresis

2016–present:Member of 2016 Beijing University Graduate Research Fund Program

Main job:The derivation of multi-wall carbon nanotubes and their major effects in separating human blood serum proteins

Publications

"Exploiture of Gel Imaging System in the Undergraduate Teaching-Designing An Integrated Experiment",China Modern Education Equipment,11/2016,pp102-103

(5)实习情况(Internship):实习经历包括申请者承担的工作、实习中的作为、对他人的积极影响及自己的收获和提升等内容。想要吸引招生人员的注意,就要从实习中收获的能力入手,巧妙地将其与所申请专业所需能力联系和统一起来,为申请成功增加更多的筹码。例如:

2016/08–present:Worked as a doctor in Bone & Joint Center of XX Hospital in XX Province which is also one of the best level hospitals

（6）获奖情况（Awards and Honors）：奖项是公信力的体现。介绍获奖情况时需要讲清楚奖项的比例、级别、颁奖单位等，注意对奖项进行筛选，有选择地列出最重要最具代表性的即可。例如，申请人多次获得过物理竞赛的奖项，有国际级、国家级、省级、市级、校级等，不用全部列出，对这些奖项进行综合考虑，选择级别较高，参与人数较多，且获奖级别相对较高的即可。例如：

2015：Second prize in the international Olympic chemistry competition

2015：National Academic Excellence Scholarship

2016：Academic Excellence Scholarship of Beijing University

除了以上内容之外，为使个人简历的内容更为丰富，还可以有选择地列出如下内容：

（7）社会实践活动（Extracurricular Activities）：课外活动、社会实践等内容在简历中的作用可大可小，可有可无。如果要写，一定要有足够的说服力，让其发挥最大的作用。与实习情况类似，申请者在活动中承担的责任、活动产生的影响以及对自身的提升等内容是必须要涉及的。例如：

Member of Publicity Department of Medicine College of Beijing University

（8）标准化考试成绩（Standard Tests）：根据所申请学校和专业的要求，如果 TOEFL、IELTS 等分数较为理想，可在简历中列出；相反，如果成绩并不理想，刚刚符合要求，则可以选择避而不谈。例如：

GRE（Oct. 2016）1280 V：470（52%），Q：800（94%），A：4.0（32%）

IBT（Aug. 2017）98 R：27，L：23，S：23，W：25

（9）兴趣爱好（Hobbies and Interests）：介绍个人兴趣爱好之前，先要确定两点，一是篇幅长度是否已经足够，二是计划列出的兴趣爱好是否与众不同，吸引读者眼球。如果兴趣爱好之外的内容已经占据了简历的过多篇幅，则可以略掉这一部分；反之，则可以用简短的语言予以介绍。兴趣爱好如果与专业相关，肯定会成为申请人专业性的加分项，而与专业并不相关却与众不同的爱好则能够体现申请人全面发展的特质，同样具有一定意义，可以简要列出。例如：

Established the Acupuncture and Massage Club of XX University

4. 反复斟酌语言，确保准确无误　个人简历写作完成后，务必认真检查，可以在自行检查之后请求他人予以协助复核。无论单词拼写、句法结构还是标点符号都要确保准确无误，因为语言上的错误会令招生人员对简历撰写人的印象大打折扣。

5. 排版干净整齐，内容一目了然　干净整洁、一目了然的简历给人以视觉享受，因此在排版时要使用正常的页边距，不要过大或过小，部分之间可以使用双倍行间距，尽量避免使用罕见字体、下划线、斜体等。排版的具体操作还应严格按照目标学校的要求。

二、个人简历范文

Basic Information

Name：Zhang Qingbin

Address：P. O. Box1708，Beijing University，Beijing，P. R. China，100875

Email:qingbin118@163. com

Tel:0086-10-6345-7896 Cell phone:0086-15012345678

Objective

Ph. D. in Orthopedics

Education

2008/09–2013/07 XX University(Ranked top 10 of China)

Major:Clinical Medicine GPA(major):3.45/4.0

Degree:Bachelor of medicine GPA(overall):3.14/4.0

2013/09–2016/07 XX University

Major:Orthopedics GPA(major):3.56/4.0

Degree:Master of Medicine GPA(overall):3.13/4.0

National Computer Rank Examination Certificate

Physicians and Physician Practicing Certificate of Qualification Certificates

Research Experience

2013/09:Was with responsibility for making preparation for the First Conference of Articular Surgery in XX Province and edited the paper for this conference

2016/02–2016/06:Gave the lessons of surgery in XX Medical College

2015/07:Was with responsibility for teaching the courses of Bone Surgery for the class of combined bachelor-master program students of grade 2016 in XX University

2015/01–2016/01:Participated in the research on SNPs in the sufferers of rheumatoid arthritis in XX Academy of Medical Sciences Publications

2014/11:Published the paper of "Avascular Necrosis of Femoral Head" in "XX Health" as the first author

2017/12:Published the paper of "Soft Tissue Balancing Techniques" for "Total Knee Arthroplasty with Severe Valgus Deformity" in "Journal of XX University" as the first author

2018/12:Will publish the paper of "Animal Experiment about Hydrazine Cross-Linking Hyaluronate Membrane Preventing Peritendon Adhesion" as the first author

2018/09:Participated in writing the monograph of "Orthopedics Operation Skills and the Precautionary Measures to Serious Errors"

Professional Experience

2016/08–present:Worked as a doctor in Bone & Joint Center of XX Hospital in XX Province which is also one of the best level hospitals

Content of work:Was in charge of patients,made the rounds of the wards,and participated in operation in emergency outpatient services

Awards and Honors

2014:Academic Excellence Scholarship of XX University

2016：Academic Excellence Scholarship of XX University

Extracurricular Activities

President of KungFu Association in XX University Special level of Club boxing and Shadowboxing

Organized the Evening Party to Welcome New Students in 2015 and 2016

Standard Tests

GRE（Oct. 2016）1280 V：470（52%），Q：800（94%），A：4.0（32%）

IBT（Aug. 2017）98 R：27，L：23，S：23，W：25

Signature：　　　　　　　　　　　　　　　　　　　　Date：

（曲㭎）

第三节　推　荐　信

优秀的推荐信（Recommendation Letter）不仅能够帮助求职者获得一份期待中的工作，对于留学申请人获得录取资格同样具有重要意义。因此，在留学文书中，推荐信的作用和地位同样不容忽视。尽管学业成绩、个人陈述、个人简历等材料才是申请海外留学深造的最重要内容，但一封精彩的推荐信能够成功地弥补上述内容中的缺陷和不足。推荐信应向招生委员会提供留学申请的其他内容未能涵盖的信息，是从旁观者的角度对申请人各方面的详细论述，包括个人素质、学业成绩和其他方面成就，以及可使申请人脱颖而出的其他经历。这些内容能够证实申请人将成为所申请的留学专业和项目的最佳人选。

一、推荐信写作注意事项

1. 推荐人的选择　尽管推荐信是从旁观者的角度对申请人进行评价，其实通常还是由申请人自己以第三人称撰写，再请推荐人签字确认。也就是说，推荐信的写作同样需要申请人自己完成。但是，在写作之前首先要确定推荐人名单。一般来讲，申请学校不会对推荐人的身份提出具体要求。因此，在读学校的校长、教授、辅导员、实习单位领导等都是比较合适的可供选择的推荐人。当然，一般的学校或专业都要求有学术推荐信，因此选择推荐人时可以重点考虑学科或专业带头人、教授、系主任等更有说服力，话语更有分量的人。但是，很多学校会要求申请人在表格中填写与推荐人的认识时间、途径、熟悉程度等内容，以确保推荐人了解和熟悉申请人。也就是说，并不是推荐人的地位越高、学术成绩越卓越就越好，而是应该选择自己较为熟悉，对自己有较多了解的人作推荐人。

2. 推荐信的内容组成　推荐信也没有统一固定的格式，但是通常包含学术成就、课外成就和个人品质三个方面的内容。

（1）学术成就（Academic Achievement）：学术成就是申请人学习能力的体现。例如：研究能力、逻辑思考和推理能力、沟通表达能力、学习主动性、科学的学习方法、智力水平与创

新能力等。撰写推荐信时要尽可能发掘自己身上的闪光点,描述时要重点突出。例如:

In my course, Sun Ce demonstrated his understanding of the theory at a good level, grasping the gist of ideas quickly and adeptly applying them in real situation. In class, he actively answered my question and raised his own opinions. From his homework, I could feel that his ideas were well founded on a basis of abundant data and materials and presented in a clear, logical and pleasant-to-read format. Sometimes he would consult me during the course of writing a paper and I could see his mind at working, digesting the information I gave him and analyzing their implications.

(2) 课外成就(Extracurricular Accomplishments): 课外成就是指学校的学习和研究之外的内容,例如实习经历、社会实践活动、比赛和获奖经历等。在这些经历中,申请人除了取得一定的成绩之外,也必定会提升个人的工作能力,包括领导能力、组织协调能力、团队协作精神等。认真梳理自己的经历,选择最触动人的内容进行合理编排,使这一部分成为推荐信中的一个亮点。例如:

She was also a good announcer and journalist with the college broadcasting station. The program she hosted was much to the liking of students audience. I am proud of her performance and amazed at her literary quality. Besides, she also displayed a high degree of leadership ability and strong work ethics. She worked very well independently and also had remarkable patience and ability to compromise in a group setting.

(3) 个人品质(Personal Qualities and Character): 如果说学术成就和课外成就更多地展示申请人的"做事"能力,那么个人品质部分重点说明申请人的"做人"情况。国外的学校希望招收素质全面、有发展前途的学生。因此,推荐信中要描述申请人的品行和特质,同样要重点突出,选择最独特的方面予以说明,不必面面俱到。例如:

Energetic and inquisitive, diligent and clever, she was also modest, always willing to listen to what others had to say. Because of these qualities, she won the trust and admiration of her friends and classmates.

3. 推荐信的结构

推荐人姓名 recommender

推荐人职位 position

联系方式(电话、邮箱、地址)corresponding information

日期 date

称谓 appellation

开头 introduction

正文 body

结尾 conclusion

推荐人签名 signature

实际上,推荐信相当于一篇议论文,分为提出论点、举例证明、重申论点三个步骤。推荐信的开头、正文和结尾分别对应这三个步骤。开头要提出论点,即对申请人的优点进行概述,正文要给出有说服力的例子作为论据以支持和证明论点,结尾再次总结申请人的优势和亮点。

二、推荐信写作原则

1. 一气呵成,前后呼应 一封优秀的推荐信应该让人在阅读时有一气呵成的感觉,篇章连贯,段落之间过渡自然,整篇文章前后呼应。

2. 逻辑鲜明,过渡自然 推荐信的语句之间要有逻辑性是最基本的写作要求,然而这也是一个难点,也很容易出现问题。写作中,很多申请人忙于罗列丰富的内容,往往忽视这些内容之间必要的逻辑关系。这一点可以在撰写完成后进行复查时重点关注,注意使用恰当的表示过渡的词、短语、句子和段落,理顺语句之间的逻辑关系。

3. 简明扼要,控制篇幅 简洁是英语写作中的另一个重要原则。一般来讲,以英语为母语或能够熟练运用英语的人写作时会使用较为精炼的语言。因此,推荐信完成后,可以请以英语为母语的朋友帮助修改,删掉不必要的内容,如果有可能,建议尽量将篇幅控制在500词左右,不宜过长。

三、推荐信范文

William Zhang

Director of English literature

Williamzhang123@126. com

Dec. 23 , 2017

Dear Sir or Madam:

Miss Anna Liu has left me a very deep impression for her zeal and earnest in Clinical Medicine studies. I am very glad to write this letter of recommendation for her because as her teacher and also as director of her college , I know very well her change from dislike and unfamiliarity to ardent love for Clinical Medicine.

I remember she was interested in economics when she first entered university because she was highly gifted in mathematics , ranking first in college entrance examination. She was first repulsive to medicine due to lack of understanding. But after just a semester , she soon became greatly interested in the specialty. Though a first-year student , she soon acquired a penetrating comprehension and stood out as one of my best undergraduates in all my years of teaching experience.

As a second-year student , guided and encouraged by teachers returning from abroad in our department , she made up her mind to further her studies in the United States and exerted herself for this sake. She attended many professional medical forums and even observed post graduated curricula. Apart from reading reference books with all earnest , she was well read in relevant Western professional books and academic papers , immensely substantiating her knowledge. This was clearly visible from her theses and perceivable from our routine communication.

At present , she is a member of our research team for a project on the AAV and gene therapy for liver cancer. So far Miss Liu has done important work for the progress of the project. To be more efficient, she in fact often lives in the lab for several days. Touched by the dedication of this young colleague, I sometimes urged her to take more rest. Miss Liu assured me that she is well aware how valuable time is for research. "I'm trying to learn as much as possible," she said, "while I'm still young and can learn things fast."

In addition, Miss Liu was also a good announcer and journalist with the college broadcasting station. "Health and Fitness", the program she hosted was much to the liking of students audience. I am proud of her performance and amazed at her literary quality. I cherish great hope that such a good student would receive better education because this would expedite the advancement of China's relevant faculty and public health.

As a professor, I greatly appreciate such an energetic and inquisitive, diligent and clever student. When she told me her desire to study abroad, I expressed full support and encouraged her to work hard for her goal. As a college director, I hereby recommend her to you with pride and pledge that she will bring your university a new refreshing atmosphere of researches. I hope you will lend her a helping hand with her application.

Signature:

练习

1. 下面是申请留学时招生委员会常要求回答的问题。请认真阅读, 尝试运用本章所学的知识, 根据自己的实际情况写一篇个人陈述。

（1）Please state your reasons for pursuing graduate study and the strengths and weaknesses of your preparation for graduate study in your proposed field. Limit your answer to one page.

（2）Please tell us your reasons for applying for graduate study, your particular area of specialization within your field of study, your professional career plans, and any additional information that you want the admissions committee to know. Your answer should not be longer than two pages.

（3）Please submit a statement of your academic and future career plans as they relate to the field which you wish to study. Your statement may not exceed 1,000 words.

（4）What are the most important qualities of you that you are hoping the admissions committee to know about?

（5）What has been your most important achievement up to now?

（6）What are your main interests outside your school study?

（7）Please describe a significant working experience that you have had.

（8）Other than your ideal job, what other careers have you considered?

（9）What is your strongest personality trait? What traits would you like to change mostly?

（10）Please account for one or two of your great academic accomplishments.

（11）What do you see as the gaps or flaws in your application, and would you like your essay to address these?

（12）What is it about your target institution that particularly interests you?

（13）Do you feel you have contributed to the life of your fellow students or the university as a whole? How?

（14）Think about what is important to you. What do you want to do with your life and how are you going to make this happen?

（15）What is the biggest challenge you have faced and how did you overcome it?

（16）What are you passionate about the subject you are applying for at postgraduate level?

（17）What areas of your major particularly motivate you?

2. 下面是一则个人陈述，请按照逻辑顺序重新排列段落。

（1）The rewards of medical research lie in its practical application, and there is no better place to observe the miracle of life than in the NICU. Each day, newborns struggle to survive, illustrating the inherent advancements and limitations of medicine. I have witnessed preemies, from 24 weeks of gestation and on, live and die. Exposure to patients revealed that people are much more than collections of cells and organs—we all share the special gift of life. My role in helping to care for them abounded with both challenge and joy.

（2）Medicine appeals to my deep appreciation for human life, inculcated by studying man as both a human being and biological machine. The decision to practice stems from a perpetual fascination with science combined with this basic love for life. I grew up capturing insects and watching PBS, always questioning the complexities of how the body works. Through academics and medical research, I have begun to answer this question.

（3）When a pod of 55 pilot whales recently beached themselves on a stretch of Cape Cod, vacationers and beach-goers came to the rescue. By high tide, they managed to save 46 whales. In explaining his motivation for jumping in to help, one volunteer simply answered, "Life." The same purpose inspires my ambition to become a physician.

（4）My passion for knowledge of the inner workings of the human body led to proactive involvement in medical research, enriching my view of medicine as well as nurturing the desire to continue research endeavors throughout my medical career. For the past two years, I have studied the relationship between structural damage and preserved clinical function in multiple sclerosis patients through functional MRI, under the tutelage of Dr. Cranston and Dr. Mahoney. Although unsure how these two factors correlate, we hypothesize that a critical period exists when the brain undergoes reorganization. In a concurrent study, I am investigating the role of the pelvic veins in cryptogenic stroke, funded through a grant awarded by the American Heart Association. The objective is to determine, via MRV, whether the pelvic veins are the source of thrombolytic emboli in cryptogenic stroke patients who also harbor a patent foramen ovale. The results of these studies not only will contribute to the advancement of medicine, but may also hold therapeutic benefits for those afflicted with such neurological damage.

(5) Reflecting on my experiences, I realize that the practice of medicine entails more than remembering and dispensing scientific facts. It requires exercising both mind and heart, along with a genuine respect for life. Baby S and my other NICU patients instilled in me a sense of how precious life is, and I am certain that my current EMT training and planned medical mission to southeast Asia will reaffirm my conviction to improve the lives of others.

(6) The career of a physician will allow me to balance an intellectual curiosity with my desire to help those in need. By helping man at his best and his worst, combining a passion for life with the pursuit of scientific knowledge, I can help heal and comfort others. I eagerly anticipate a vocation in which my patients fuel my search for knowledge, and that search embodies reciprocal benefits to my patients. When asked why I have chosen a medical career, I can confidently respond, "Life."

(7) My first patient, Baby S, arrived nine weeks prematurely and spent the first month of life in the NICU. Due to the presence of an extrachromosomal fragment, he suffered slight mental retardation. His mother, who had the same condition, visited infrequently during his hospital stay. When she did, her visits were brief and inattentive. I grew quite fond of Baby S, often watching him snuggle into the blankets like a small burrito. Although his sky blue eyes moved in a spastic manner, they gave life to his somewhat immobile body. He rarely showed signs of discomfort, whether hungry or needing a change. I tried to give him the extra attention he lacked. At times, he rewarded my efforts to interact with a smile; other times, he gave me a dirty diaper.

3. 假设你研究生毕业后有出国继续深造的计划，请自拟一份个人简历。

下篇
英文医学论文写作中的语言运用

第一章 常用词汇

在英文医学论文的写作过程中,困难常源于不能准确掌握核心词汇的意义和用法,不会使用连接词和修饰词。在日常写作中,一方面要注意积累医学专业方面的常用词汇,另一方面要用心学习写作中常用关键词的用法。本章总结了医学论文写作过程中的核心词汇,并根据写作内容做了分类,配以例句,以期从例句和日常阅读中更好地掌握词语,从而提高论文的写作质量。

第一节 论文写作常用词汇

为了便于学习和使用,本部分词汇共分 12 类。

一、描写研究课题的意义及重要性

本部分词汇主要用于描写研究课题的意义和重要性,常用于 Introduction 和 Discussion 的写作中。

- **associate**

Overexpression of PKCβ2 dominant-negative mutant did not *associate* with Rb.

过度表达 PKCβ2 显性负性突变体与 Rb 蛋白的表达无相关性。

- **consist of**

Macrovascular complications in diabetic patients *consist* mainly *of* cardiovascular events.

糖尿病患者的大血管并发症主要包括心血管疾病。

- **involve**

Analyses concerning lung cancer reliability did not *involve* statistical tests because of the small sample size.

因为样本量过小,不使用统计分析方法分析肺癌可信度。

- **participate**

All residents working on the ICU were considered eligible to *participate* in the study.

所有在 ICU 工作的住院医师都有资格参与这项研究。

二、描述某个领域的现状或研究计划

本部分词汇主要用于描述某个领域的研究现状或研究计划,常用于 Introduction 和

Discussion 的写作中。

- **characterize**

This study sought to *characterize* sinus rhythm left atrial ECG patterns and their relationship to parasympathetic responses.

本研究旨在分析窦性节律下左房心电图的特征及它们与迷走反应的关系。

- **demonstrate**

Preterm infants with bronchopulmonary dysplasia often *demonstrate* sucking difficulties.

支气管肺发育不良的早产儿常出现吮吸困难。

- **elucidate**

Additional studies are warranted to *elucidate* the functional significance of KIR genes associated with treatment outcomes.

还需要进行进一步的研究以明确 KIR 基因的功能意义及其相关的治疗效果。

- **establish**

BTICs can *establish* GBMs at the clonal level and perpetuate across serial transplantation.

脑肿瘤起始细胞能够再生出同源的恶性胶质瘤,并且在多次传代后仍保留此种能力。

- **identify**

A 24-hour ECG record may *identify* those most at risk from sudden death from dysrhythmia.

24 小时心电图监测可以确定哪些患者最有可能出现心律失常,并导致猝死。

- **investigate**

The suction skin blister method has potential as a diagnostic tool to *investigate* small fiber neuropathies.

抽吸皮肤水疱法有可能作为研究小纤维神经病变的诊断手段。

- **monitor**

The distal catheter opening was positioned within the neobladder reservoir to *monitor* pouch pressures.

导管末端开口置于新膀胱,以便观察新膀胱压力变化。

三、描述需要解决的问题

本部分词汇主要用于描述需要解决的问题,常用于 Introduction 的写作中。

- **address**

Our study could not *address* this pathogenic question.

我们的研究无法解释这个致病机制问题。

- **approach**

A convenient *approach* to most anemias that result from production defects is to examine cellular changes.

对大多数因生成不足所致的贫血来说,合适的处理方法是检查血细胞的变化。

- **in contrast**

In contrast, cortical anillin accumulates normally in myosin-depleted embryos.

相反,在无肌球蛋白的胚胎中,皮层苯胺素集聚正常。

- **represent**

In many tumors, the banding patterns *represent* complete methylation.

在很多肿瘤中,染色体带型表现出完全的甲基化。

四、表达过去和现在的时间

本部分主要是关于过去和现在时间的词汇,常用于 Introduction 和 Discussion 的写作中。

- **current**

The *current* immunosuppressive regimen includes cyclosporine.

现行的免疫抑制治疗方案包括环孢素。

- **previous**

Previous studies describe a correlation between proliferation and cell survival.

以前的研究描述了增殖与细胞存活之间的相关性。

- **recent**

Our conclusions are generally consistent with several other *recent* reviews.

我们的结论与最近的其他几个综述基本一致。

- **to date**

To date, the mechanism of pathogenesis is not fully understood.

迄今为止,尚未完全阐明其致病机制。

五、举例

本部分词汇主要用于举例,经常用于 Introduction,Results 和 Discussion 的写作中。

- **especially**

Dementia is a condition of declining mental abilities, *especially* memory.

老年性痴呆是指脑功能下降的一种状态,特别是记忆力下降。

- **include**

Hypersensitivity reactions, *including* systemic anaphylaxis, are common.

过敏反应,包括全身性过敏反应,是非常普遍的。

- **in particular/particularly**

In particular/Particularly, asthma and chronic obstructive pulmonary disease(COPD)both overlap and converge in older people.

哮喘与慢性阻塞性肺疾病常同时发生且集中发病,在老年人群中尤为如此。

六、描述实验过程

本部分词汇主要用于描述实验过程，常用于 Methods 的写作中。

- **acquire**

Generalized-onset seizures that *acquire* focal features are easily misdiagnosed as complex partial.

伴有局部症状的全身发作性癫痫发作很容易被误诊为复杂的部分性发作。

- **afford**

The resolution of a complicating cystitis will usually *afford* some relief.

消除并发的膀胱炎通常可以减轻一些症状。

- **assess**

Antibodies to actin were used to *assess* loading.

抗肌动蛋白抗体用于衡量上样量。

- **conduct**

The muscle fibers then conduct signals in the same way that nerve fibers *conduct* them.

然后肌纤维也像神经纤维一样传导信号。

- **furnish**

The well-being of each individual cell is dependent on the adequacy of its environment to *furnish* nutrition and carry away metabolites.

每个细胞的健康有赖于周围环境充分供应营养并运走代谢产物。

- **generate**

Alternative adherent cell cultures can now *generate* higher cell densities with less labor.

现在选择黏附细胞培养法可以用更少的劳动培育更高密度细胞。

- **perform**

Cells are organized into tissues that *perform* specific functions.

细胞构成组织，并发挥着特殊的功能。

- **proceed**

If imaging is normal, one should *proceed* at once with vigorous antihypertensive therapy.

如果成像正常，应立即开始积极的抗高血压治疗。

- **subject to**

The incoming amino acids are *subject to* transamination with α-ketoglutarate, to yield glutamate.

进入肝的氨基酸可与 α-酮戊二酸进行转氨作用，产生谷氨酸。

- **undertake**

We aimed to *undertake* an integrated analysis of a complete human genome in a clinical context.

该研究旨在从临床角度对完整的人体基因组信息进行整合分析。

七、描述先后顺序

本部分词汇主要用于描述先后顺序,常用于 Methods 的写作中。

● immediate

It requires *immediate* treatment with steroid replacement.

需立即用类固醇替代疗法。

● instant

Generally speaking, gene transcriptions are temporally and spatially regulated in response to *instant* environmental and inner status.

一般来说,基因转录是受时空调控的以适应当时的外部环境和自身内环境的影响。

● in the course of/during the course of

Substantial activation of platelets can occur *in the course of* hemodialysis.

在透析过程中,患者的大部分血小板存在着活性。

Significantly more obese and hypertensive participants developed diabetes *during the course of* the study.

在研究过程中,肥胖或高血压的受试者发生糖尿病的概率更大。

● simultaneous

Every patient with gonorrhea should be checked to exclude *simultaneous* syphilis and HIV infection.

每位淋病患者应接受检查以排除并发梅毒和艾滋病感染。

● subsequent

The possibility of *subsequent* cervical cancer is thus absolutely prevented.

因此,日后发生宫颈癌的可能性得以绝对防止。

八、描述实验结果

本部分词汇主要用于描述实验结果,常用于 Results 和 Discussion 的写作中。

1. 降低、减少,抑制、阻止

● decrease

However, this *decrease* was accompanied by a corresponding *decrease* in dGTP concentrations.

但是,这个降低伴随着 dGTP 浓度的相应降低。

● hamper

In addition, squamous metaplasia and loss of ciliary coordination further *hamper* antibacterial defenses.

此外,鳞状细胞转化以及纤毛协调作用丧失进一步损害抗菌性防御机制。

● **inhibit**

Other prostaglandins can *inhibit* certain of the processes of inflammation.

另一些前列腺素可抑制炎症的某些过程。

● **reduce**

Anti-inflammatory agents are topical agents that *reduce* inflammation.

消炎药是局部用药,可以消除炎症。

● **suppress**

Intraoperative stress may *suppress* the adaptive immune system.

手术应激可以抑制适应性免疫系统。

2. 提高、增加、激活

● **elevate**

Metabolic actions: epinephrine and isoproterenol *elevate* blood glucose by glycogenolysis, and by inhibiting glucose utilization.

代谢的作用:通过糖元分解并抑制对葡萄糖的利用,肾上腺素和异丙肾上腺素可以提高血糖浓度。

● **enhance**

Imiquimod did not *enhance* DNA repair in skin organ cultures.

在皮肤组织器官培养中咪喹莫特没有促进 DNA 修复。

● **increase**

Numerous microvilli *increase* the canalicular surface area.

无数的微绒毛增加了管道的表面积。

● **raise**

A history of primary tumors elsewhere should immediately *raise* this suspicion.

其他任何部位有原发性肿瘤病史时,应立即提出怀疑。

● **stimulate**

Some tumors metastatic in bone *stimulate* excessive new bone formation.

有些骨的转移瘤可刺激大量新骨形成。

3. 其他词汇

● **alter**

Drugs may *alter* the protein binding of other agents.

有些药物可以改变另一些药物的蛋白结合。

● **confirm**

Further prospective studies are needed to *confirm* these associations.

但尚需进一步的前瞻性研究来证实这些关联。

● **determine**

Appropriate studies should readily *determine* the cause.

进行适当的检查可以明确诊断病因。

- **distinguish**

The isolation of RSV helps *distinguish* bronchiolitis from asthma.

呼吸道合胞病毒的分离有助于区别毛细支气管炎和支气管哮喘。

- **exert**

Antimicrobial agents *exert* their effects by four different mechanisms.

抗微生物药物通过四种不同的机制来发挥作用。

- **exhibit**

In addition, these mice *exhibit* reduced metabolism and body temperature.

此外,这些小鼠的代谢和体温下降。

- **illustrate**

Positive samples clearly *illustrate* the sensitivity of FIAX testing and its reliability for screening serum samples.

阳性标本清楚地表明 FIAX 试验的敏感性及其用于筛选血清标本的可靠性。

- **manipulate**

Recent reports suggest that tumor viruses such as EBV and KSHV *manipulate* the tumor microenvironment through the secretion of specific viral and cellular components into exosomes.

近期的报道提示,EBV、KSHV 等肿瘤病毒通过外泌体来调节肿瘤的微环境。

- **mediate**

Mediate percussion is more popular.

间接叩诊更为常用。

Cholinergic fiber *mediate* eccrine sweat secretion.

胆碱能纤维调节外泌汗腺的分泌。

- **modulate**

In addition, MSCs can reprogram kidney cell differentiation, and *modulate* neo-kidney transplantation in CRF.

此外,MSC 可以重新调整肾脏细胞分化,调节 CRF 中的新肾移植。

- **retain**

Balancing this, however, such lines usually *retain* very low activity levels for some essential hepatocyte functions.

不过,通过平衡这种扩张潜能,这种细胞系通常保持非常低的活动水平,以保持某些必需的肝细胞功能。

九、讨论和介绍实验意义

本部分词汇主要用于介绍和讨论实验意义,常用于 Discussion 部分。

1. 可能、猜测、好像

- **assume**

According to the nature of the pathologic process, skin lesions *assume* more or less distinct characteristics.

根据病理过程的性质,皮肤损害或多或少地表现出独特的特征。

- **presume/presumably**

We *presume* that the polymer used in the group D plates had more ductile properties.

我们推测 D 组固定板的聚合物更具延展性。

Presumably, maternal immunity reduces the virulence of the fetal infection.

可以推测,母体免疫力能够降低胎儿感染的毒性。

- **speculative**

The mechanisms by which diabetes and high glucose concentrations activate the oxidase remain *speculative*.

糖尿病和高糖活化氧化酶的机制仍然未知。

- **suppose**

It would seem reasonable to *suppose* that the deep glands are set in action reflexly, though of this there is no proof.

人们认为深层腺体的活动是反射性的。这似乎有道理,尽管尚未得到证明。

2. 其他词汇

- **accompany**

Hypertension and thrombosis *accompany* arteriosclerosis and atherosclerosis.

动脉硬化和动脉粥样硬化时会出现高血压和血栓。

- **anticipate**

With the aid of HBsAg quantitation, it appears that we can *anticipate* an individualized approach to tailoring the treatment duration.

借助 HBsAg 定量,我们预期可以通过个性化的方法来调整疗程。

- **attribute**

We *attribute* this result to the quality of the antibodies used in both studies.

我们能够得到这些结果是因为两项研究所用的抗体质量较高。

- **conceive**

Patients who did *conceive* were taken off DHEA supplementation once a normal rise in pregnancy hormone was observed over two measurements.

一旦观察到妊娠患者的孕激素正常地升高至 2 倍以上,停用 DHEA。

- **hypothesize**

We *hypothesize* that cellular adhesion may play an important role in the differentiation response of the ASC.

我们推测,细胞黏附在脂肪干细胞的分化过程中发挥了重要作用。

- **in the presence of/in the absence of**

They fix complement well *in the presence of* antigen.

它们在与抗原结合后易固定补体。

The enhancement of injury thus occurs *in the absence of* elevation of temperature.

这种损害加重的现象同样发生在体温没有升高的情况下。

- **indicate**

When local health authorities *indicate* that influenza activity is present in the community, the etiology of an acute febrile respiratory illness can be attributed to influenza with a high degree of certainty, particularly if the typical features of abrupt onset and systemic symptoms are present.

当地方卫生部门提示在该地区发生流感时,如果出现突然发生全身症状的典型特征,即可相当肯定地将急性发热性呼吸道疾病诊断为流感。

- **insight**

Each new *insight* into the pathophysiology of malignant transformation has provided new targets for therapy.

对恶变的病理生理学的每一个新认识都为治疗提出了新的目标。

- **notion**

These data support the *notion* that the mechanism underlying WRF is important in determining its prognostic significance.

这些数据说明,WRF 的内在机制对决定预后有重要意义。

- **shed light on**

Advances in neuroimaging, electrophysiology, and prospective behavioral testing have *shed light on* how epileptic seizures disrupt the consciousness system.

神经影像学、电生理学和潜在行为测试的进展揭示了癫痫发作如何破坏意识系统。

十、比较

本部分词汇主要用于比较,常用于 Results 和 Discussion 的写作中。

- **compare**

We sought to *compare* vaccine interventions for poliomyelitis outbreak control.

我们试图对控制脊髓灰质炎暴发的疫苗进行干预比较。

- **consistent with**

Our conclusions are generally *consistent with* several other recent reviews.

我们的结论与其他几个最近的综述基本一致。

- **equivalent**

An *equivalent* volume of saline was added to another 1.5ml blood sample to serve as control.

等量的生理盐水加入到另一份 1.5ml 的血液样本中,作为对照。

- **fold**

E-cadherin mRNA and protein were increased 4-*fold* and 4.3-*fold*, as well as albumin mRNA and protein 5-*fold* and 3.3-*fold*, respectively.

细胞钙黏蛋白 mRNA 水平升高 4 倍,蛋白升高 4.3 倍;白蛋白 mRNA 水平升高 5 倍,蛋白升高 3.3 倍。

- **in line with**

The BP targets should be *in line with* those recommended for patients with diabetic renal disease.

降压的目标值应与糖尿病、肾病推荐的降压目标值相同。

- **resemble**

Chronic gout, particularly if widespread, may *resemble* rheumatoid or osteoarthritis.

慢性痛风,特别是病变广泛时,与类风湿或骨关节炎类似。

- **versus**

The effectiveness of concurrent *versus* sequential regimens is not known.

同期(用药)方案与序贯(用药)方案两者相比的有效性尚不清楚。

十一、常用修饰词

本部分是一些常用的修饰词。

- **approximately**

Angioplasty produced clinically worthwhile improvement for *approximately* 50% of patients.

血管成形术可使 50% 的患者明显改善临床症状。

- **compelling**

Here, we provide *compelling* genetic evidence that calpain is required for LTP.

本研究中,我们提供了翔实的基因证据证明钙蛋白酶为 LTP 所必需。

- **dramatic**

Although results from PSO are *dramatic*, the postoperative thoracic subcurve remains significantly different from normal.

尽管从椎弓根截骨术得到的结果引人注目,但术后胸椎亚曲线分析仍明显不同于正常人群。

- **exclusively**

Four surgeons used the transcallosal approach *exclusively*, and three surgeons used the endoscopic approach *exclusively*.

四位医生仅采用经胼胝体入路手术,三位医生仅用内窥镜入路手术。

- **extensively**

Currently the most *extensively* studied gene is apolipoprotein E.

当前研究最为广泛的基因是载脂蛋白 E。

- **permanently**

We report on the finished genome sequence of *Carnobacterium* sp. 17-4, which has been isolated from *permanently* cold sea water.

我们报告了肉毒杆菌 17-4 的已完成的基因组序列。该菌从持续低温海水中分离出来。

- **potentially**

Meningitis remains a *potentially* devastating disease.

脑膜炎仍然是潜在的致命性疾病。

- **predominantly**

It is not understood why the cord is *predominantly* affected.

目前尚不清楚脊髓成为主要受累部位的原因。

- **radically**

We wish to put forward a *radically* different structure for the salt of deoxyribose nucleic acid.

我们想对 DNA 盐提出一种根本不同的结构。

- **spontaneously**

The myocardium will contract *spontaneously* without any nerve supply.

在没有神经支配的情况下,心肌仍可自发收缩。

十二、常见易混词

本部分是一些常见的易混词语,需要注意区分。

- **alternate, alternative**

alternate 交替的,轮流的;alternative 另外的,选择的。

The molecule doesn't contain *alternate* single and double bonds,这种分子不含交替的单双键。

An *alternative* treatment is GM-CSF injections.

可替代的治疗方案为注射 GM-CSF。

- **compose, consist, comprise**

compose 意为"组成,构成",是及物动词,一般用 be composed of 的形式。例如:A single muscle is *composed* of thousands of fibers. 一块肌肉由成千上万的肌纤维构成。

consist 意为"由……组成",是不及物动词,一般用 consist of 的形式。例如:Taste buds *consist* of four different cell types. 味蕾有四种不同的细胞类型。

comprise "包括",也有"由……组成"的意思。例如:The hallmarks of cancer *comprise* six biological capabilities acquired during the multistep development of human tumors. 恶性肿瘤的功能特征包含六种生物学能力,是人类肿瘤在多步骤发展的过程中逐步获得的。

- **conserved, conservative**

conserved 保存的,保持的;conservative 保守的,守旧的。

The primary outcome was local recurrence in the *conserved* breast.

主要结果为保留乳腺侧的局部复发。

Most authors reported favorable results after *conservative* management.

大多数学者报道,保守治疗可以取得理想结果。

● **continual, continuous**

continual 经常发生的,不断的;continuous 连续的,不间断的。

With *continual* improvements in immunosuppression and medical management, technical achievements, and improvements in procurement and preservation, patient survival rate has been improved steadily.

由于免疫抑制和医疗方案、技术成果以及获取与保存技术的不断改进,患者的生存率稳步提高。

The common symptom to all the types is *continuous* hoarseness.

所有类型的喉炎都表现出持续性声嘶的常见症状。

● **diminish, decrease**

diminish 削弱,减到很少;decrease 减少,并不一定减到很少。

The degree of fatty change in the liver tends to *diminish* as the disease progresses.

肝脂肪变的程度往往随着疾病的进展而减轻。

Sweating helps to *decrease* body temperature.

发汗有助于降低体温。

● **dramatically, drastically**

dramatically 显著地;drastically 激烈地,彻底地。

The management of thoracic vascular injury has improved *dramatically* over the past two decades.

在过去 20 年中,胸动脉损伤的治疗手段进步非常显著。

The mattress suture *drastically* reduces the need for scoring (with its inherent problems of weakness) and the need for cartilage grafting.

褥式缝合彻底减少了软骨刻痕的应用(其固有的弱化软骨的问题)和软骨移植的需要。

● **minimal, trivial**

minimal 最小的;trivial 轻微的,不重要的。

Apart from *minimal* bleeding, no other complication was encountered.

除了少量的出血外,没有发现其他并发症。

Burns can be as *trivial* as a simple cut, or can be cause for real concern.

烧伤可能与小创伤一样无关紧要,也可能十分值得关注。

● **provided that, providing**

provided that 假如,可以连接句子;providing 提供,是现在分词。

Provided that fetal heart can be heard at a normal rate, no interference should be contemplated for fetal distress.

倘若能听到胎儿心率正常,就不应该认为出现胎儿窘迫而进行手术。

The history is most important in *providing* information regarding the etiology of diarrhea.

病史能够为确定腹泻的病因提供极为重要的线索。

- **use,using,utilize,employ**

写作时经常会使用 use。若用 using 导致与主句的主语名词不一致时,可用 with 或 by 取代。

Using specific assays, Matrix proteins were analyzed.

宜改为:Matrix proteins were analyzed *with* specific assays.

采用特异性的检测方法来分析基质蛋白。

utilize 意为"利用,有效使用",与 use 不同,不能相互替代。

Cells utilize mainly fats and proteins to supply their energy needs.

细胞主要利用脂肪和蛋白质来满足它们的能量需要。

employ 意为"雇用,使从事于",也可表示采用某种方法或手段。

Many hospitals now *employ* fetal monitoring during labour.

目前许多医院在分娩时进行胎儿监测。

- **vary,change**

vary 意为"变化,改变",侧重于不同;change 意为"变化,改变",强调变化。

The neurologic manifestations of neuroblastoma *vary* considerably.

成神经细胞瘤的神经系统表现变异很大。

Measures to *change* this are desperately needed.

亟待采取措施来改变这一现状。

（刘晓燕）

第二节　词汇的误用

一、名词误用

1. 单复数误用

例 1　误:Prostate cancer is the most common cancer diagnosed in men and one of the leading causes of cancer death.

分析:death 意为"生命的终止,死亡状态"时,是抽象不可数名词。意为"死,死亡"时,为可数名词。此处用法属于后者,因此改用复数。

正:Prostate cancer is the most common cancer diagnosed in men and one of the leading causes of cancer deaths.

译文:前列腺癌是男性最常见的癌症,也是癌症致死的主要原因之一。

例 2　误：Phytoene synthase from the <u>bacteria</u> Erwinia uredovora（crtB）has been overexpressed in tomato.

分析：名词作定语时一般用单数，除非本身就以复数概念出现，例如，"结果部分"用 Results section.

正：Phytoene synthase from the <u>bacterium</u> Erwinia uredovora（crtB）has been overexpressed in tomato.

译文：嗜夏孢欧文<u>菌</u>（crtB）中的八氢番茄红素合酶在番茄中过度<u>表达</u>。

2."of+ 名词"作后置定语造成行文拖沓

例 3　误：Investigators and patients were unaware of the <u>status of treatment allocation</u>.

分析：行文简洁是科技文体的特点。简化定语的方法之一是将作后置定语的介词短语中的名词提前，直接作前置定语，同时去掉介词 of。名词提前的条件是不因此产生歧义。此句中的 of treatment allocation 构成后置定语，修饰 status。将 treatment allocation 提前不会产生歧义，且行文简洁。

正：Investigators and patients were unaware of the <u>treatment allocation status</u>.

译文：研究人员和患者均不知晓<u>治疗分配情况</u>。

3. 名词堆砌

例 4　误：The culture method and the SPR method for <u>four bacteria detection</u> did not differ significantly in any respect（P>0.05）.

分析：句中 four bacteria detection 名词作前置定语导致歧义，可指"对四种细菌做的检测"或"用四种细菌做的检测"。此处 four bacteria 是 detection 的受动者，应改为"of+ 名词"作后置定语，清楚体现动宾关系，即 the detection of four bacteria。

正：The culture method and the SPR method for <u>the detection of four bacteria</u> did not differ significantly in any respect（P>0.05）.

译文：培养法和 SPR 法用于检测四种细菌时无显著差异（P>0.05）。

例 5　误：A new <u>angiogenesis balance</u> is achieved in patients after surgery.

分析：若后置定语由非 of 的其他介词引导，则不能轻易将名词提前直接作定语，否则易造成语义关系不明。本例实际上是 balance in angiogenesis（血管生成中的平衡），angiogenesis 提前导致表意不清，因此应改为后置定语。

正：A new <u>balance in angiogenesis</u> is achieved in patients after surgery.

译文：术后，患者的<u>血管生成</u>形成了新的<u>平衡</u>。

二、动词误用

1. 动词选用不当

例 6　误：Geneticists have yet to <u>analyze</u> the complex code by which epigenetic marks interact with the other components of the genome.

分析：analyze 一词意为 to separate something into its parts in order to study its nature or structure, 即指分析的过程, 并不涉及"破译"的结果, 无法表达"解码"。准确的表达应该是 decipher 或 decode, 意思为 to convert from a code or cipher to plain text。

正: Geneticists have yet to <u>decipher/decode</u> the complex code by which epigenetic marks interact with the other components of the genome.

译文: 目前, 遗传学家还未<u>破解</u>外遗传标签与基因组其他组成之间产生互动的复杂编码。

例 7 误: <u>It should also be noticed</u> that a higher number of carriers than expected was observed among patients with pancreatic cancer.

分析: 动词 notice 与 note 都表示"注意, 留意"。note 还可表示"特别提到, 指出"。例如: The judge noted that Miller had no previous criminal record. (法官指出米勒没有犯罪前科。)但从语体考虑, note 比 notice 更正式, 而且"It should be noted that..."为固定搭配, 意为"值得注意的是"。

正: <u>It should also be noted</u> that a higher number of carriers than expected was observed among patients with pancreatic cancer.

译文: <u>值得注意的是</u>, 胰腺癌患者中的携带率比预期要高。

例 8 误: Antimetabolites are analogues of natural substrates which <u>rival</u> with the natural substrate for active sites on an enzyme.

分析: rival 意为"与……相匹敌; 比得上", compete 意为"竞争"。而此处指相互竞争, 故选用后者。

正: Antimetabolites are analogues of natural substrates which <u>compete</u> with the natural substrate for active sites on an enzyme.

译文: 抗代谢物是天然底物的同类物, 能与天然底物竞争酶的活性部位。

例 9 误: Further studies are warranted to <u>affirm</u> these findings and to increase study power.

分析: affirm 意为"申明, 断言", 通常为口头保证。而在科技文体中表示"证实"多用 confirm 或 validate, 表示"(提供证据)证实"。

正: Further studies are warranted to <u>confirm</u> these findings and to increase study power.

译文: 有必要进行进一步的研究, 以确认这些调查结果并提高研究的效力。

例 10 误: Prospective observational study has been <u>done</u> as previously described.

分析: 在本句中表达"做研究"或"做某一具体的实验", 应选用语体较为正式的词, 如 perform 或 conduct, 而 do 过于口语化。

正: Prospective observational study has been <u>performed</u> as previously described.

译文: 如前所述, 已<u>进行</u>过前瞻性观察研究。

2. 动词用法有误

例 11 误: Additionally, the cognitive symptoms of depression, most notably hopelessness, <u>interfere</u> treatment participation.

分析: interfere 为不及物动词, 须加介词跟宾语。interfere with sth. 意为"干扰, 妨碍",

interfere in sth. 意为"干涉,介入"。句中表达的意思是"干扰",故应该在 interfere 后加 with。

正:Additionally, the cognitive symptoms of depression, most notably hopelessness, <u>interfere with</u> treatment participation.

译文:此外,绝望是抑郁症最显著的认知症状,会<u>干扰</u>治疗的参与。

例 12 误:The spleen is located in the middle energizer, below the diaphragm and the spleen's meridians <u>connect to</u> the stomach, <u>to which</u> it is exteriorly-interiorly related.

分析:connect 是不及物动词,与介词 with 或 to 搭配,意思稍有不同。用介词 with 指把 A 与 B 联系起来或连接在一起,A、B 之间不分主次,且其中的介词 with 也可换成连词 and;用介词 to 指把 A 连接在 B 上,其中以 B 为主,以 A 为辅。根据句意,应该在 connect 后面加 with。

正:The spleen is located in the middle energizer, below the diaphragm and the spleen's meridians <u>connect with</u> the stomach, <u>with which</u> it is exteriorly-interiorly related.

译文:脾位于中焦,膈之下,通过经络与胃<u>相连</u>,与胃相表里。

三、形容词误用

1. 形容词选用有误

例 13 误:Ectopic Notch1 activation is <u>enough</u> to inhibit Ascl1 expression and neuroblast production by astrocytes after stroke.

分析:本例误将 enough 用作形容词,enough 只能用作限定词、副词或代词。sufficient 是形容词,意为"足够的,充足的",表示"具备(达到某目的)的最低标准"。它可以作定语,也可以作表语。

正:Ectopic Notch1 activation is <u>sufficient</u> to inhibit Ascl1 expression and neuroblast production by astrocytes after stroke.

译文:异位 Notch1 激活足以抑制中风后星形胶质细胞 Ascl1 表达和成神经细胞的产生。

例 14 误:Moreover, expression of VEGF mRNA was shown to <u>be correlative to</u> vascularity in both gliomas and meningiomas.

分析:本句中 correlative 意为"紧密相关的,相互关联的",一般用作前置定语,后跟 study、data、model 等。若表达"X 与 Y 相关"可用:X correlates with Y,或 X is correlated with Y。如果表示两者呈正或负相关,可用"X is positively/negatively correlated with Y"。

正:Moreover, expression of VEGF mRNA was shown to <u>correlate with</u> vascularity in both gliomas and meningiomas.

译文:此外,VEGF 的 mRNA 表达显示和胶质瘤和脑膜瘤的血管生成都有<u>相关性</u>。

2. 复合形容词误用

例 15 误:In some <u>high risk</u> patients with delirium, coma, or shock, high-dose dexamethasone in addition to antibiotics reduces mortality.

分析:本句中 high 与 risk 构成合成形容词,修饰 patients,但两词之间缺乏起连接作用的连字符。

正：In some <u>high-risk</u> patients with delirium, coma, or shock, high-dose dexamethasone in addition to antibiotics reduces mortality.

译文：在一些并发谵妄、昏迷或休克的<u>高危</u>患者中，大剂量地塞米松与抗生素合用可降低死亡率。

四、代词误用

严格地讲，代词是代替名词，在句子中起名词的作用。代词应该与其指代的名词在单复数形式上保持一致。例如：

例16 误：Cytomegaloviruses (CMV) are typical herpesviruses both in <u>its</u> structure and mode of replication.

分析：句中的 its 指代前面复数形式的 Cytomegaloviruses，所以应将形容词性物主代词 its 改为相应的复数形式 their。

正：Cytomegaloviruses (CMV) are typical herpesviruses both in <u>their</u> structure and mode of replication.

译文：巨细胞病毒（CMV）在<u>其</u>结构和复制方式上都是典型的疱疹病毒。

五、副词误用

1. 副词选用有误

例17 误：The detection rates of metabolic syndrome in three years were 23.9%, 16.7% and 14.4% <u>separately</u> and the differences of detection rates between different genders were not statistical significance ($P>0.05$).

分析：separately 意为"单独的，分别的"，用于描述对象作为独立个体而分别存在或分离的。respectively 意为"分别的，各自的，依次的"，而句中要求用该副词体现指定出的 three years 与 23.9%、16.7% 和 14.4%，按照顺序逐一对应。因此将 separately 替换为 respectively 以表示各年数据的一一对应。

正：The detection rates of metabolic syndrome in three years were 23.9%, 16.7% and 14.4% <u>respectively</u> and the differences of detection rates between different genders were not statistical significance ($P>0.05$).

译文：三年体检资料中代谢综合征检出率<u>分别</u>为 23.9%，16.7% 和 14.4%，各年性别间检出率差异均无统计学意义（$P>0.05$）。

例18 误：FGFR3 mutations (12%) <u>usually</u> affected known kinase-activating sites.

分析：usually 意为"通常地，正常地"，强调时间间隔短；typically 指"通常，一般"，强调总是以某种方式发生，体现一种规律性。例如：The disease typically takes several weeks to appear.（这种疾病通常在几周后才表现出来。）

正：FGFR3 mutations (12%) <u>typically</u> affected known kinase-activating sites.

译文：FGFR3 突变（12%）<u>通常</u>影响已知的激酶活性位点。

例 19 误：Endostar <u>creatively</u> harbors a 9-amino-acid insert on the N-terminus of the endostatin protein.

分析：在注重客观描述的科技文体的写作中不宜使用诸如 creatively、successfully 等带有比较强烈主观色彩的副词。

正：Endostar harbors a 9-amino-acid insert on the N-terminus of the endostatin protein.

译文：恩度在内皮抑素肽链 N 端增加了一个含 9 个氨基酸的插入片段。

2. 副词误用作连词

例 20 误：This molecular biological method can detect the definite nucleic acid component of the bacterium genome, <u>thus it can</u> avoid deviations originating from phenotype changes.

分析：句中使用 thus 连接两个并列的句子，但 thus 只能作副词，不能充当连词连接并列短语或句子。因此，可以使用 thus 修饰 avoid，同时在两个并列句子间添加并列连词 and。

正：This molecular biological method can detect the definite nucleic acid component of the bacterium genome, <u>and can thus</u> avoid deviations originating from phenotype changes.

译文：这种分子生物学方法能够检测确定的细菌基因组核酸成分，<u>从而</u>可以避免表型改变引起的偏差。

例 21 误：These results suggest that *DNMT3A* is not responsible for DNA methylation in the promoter, first exon, or first intron regulatory regions of *Oct4*, <u>in addition</u>, the DNA methylation status was not correlated with the expression level of *Oct4*.

分析：介词短语 in addition 在句中作状语，不能连接并列句。因此，可将 in addition 前的逗号改成句号，将原句变为两个独立的句子，in addition 在第二个句子中充当句首状语。

正：These results suggest that *DNMT3A* is not responsible for DNA methylation in the promoter, first exon, or first intron regulatory regions of *Oct4*. <u>In addition</u>, the DNA methylation status was not correlated with the expression level of *Oct4*.

译文：这些结果表明，*DNMT3A* 与 *Oct4* 基因启动子，第一外显子或第一内含子调控区域的 DNA 甲基化不相关。<u>此外</u>，DNA 甲基化的程度与 *Oct4* 基因的表达水平不相关。

六、冠词误用

1. 定冠词 the 的误用

例 22 误：CT scanning can also provide additional other valuable information, especially on location and extent of hemorrhage.

分析：由于汉语中不存在冠词，在英语表达时经常会出现冠词的误用或不恰当省略，本句中特指"出血部位和范围"，因此前面应该加定冠词 the。

正：CT scanning can also provide additional other valuable information, especially on <u>the</u> location and extent of hemorrhage.

译文：电子计算机断层扫描检查还能提供额外的有价值的资料，特别是关于出血部位和范围。

例 23 误：We drew <u>the</u> similar conclusion that many genes are associated with the pathophysiology and outcome following TBI.

分析：句中 similar conclusion 表示"一个相似的结论"，并非特指，因此不用定冠词 the，应改为不定冠词 a。

正：We drew <u>a</u> similar conclusion that many genes are associated with the pathophysiology and outcome following TBI.

译文：我们得到<u>一个相似的结论</u>：许多基因和脑外伤病理生理改变和预后有关。

例 24 误：Single-stranded cDNA was synthesized using M-MLV reverse transcriptase.

分析：句中 M-MLV reverse transcriptase 是一种实验材料，通常固定的实验方法或特指的实验材料前要加定冠词。

正：Single-stranded cDNA was synthesized using <u>the</u> M-MLV reverse transcriptase.

译文：用 M-MLV 逆转录酶合成单链 cDNA。

2. 不定冠词 a/an 的误用

例 25 误：This results in <u>aberrant gene expression profile</u> in many kinds of cancers.

分析：profile 作"表达谱"讲，为可数名词，单数形式时前面必须加冠词，此处非特指，因此应该使用不定冠词 an。

正：This results in <u>an aberrant gene expression profile</u> in many kinds of cancers.

译文：这导致在多种癌症中产生<u>异常基因表达谱</u>。

例 26 误：HPV-positive cervical cancer cells with a higher level of *Oct4* also had <u>stronger colony-forming ability</u> than did HPV-negative cervical cancer cells.

分析：ability 表示抽象意义的"能力"时，为不可数名词。例如：He is a man of ability.（他是位有能力的人。）若表示"有能力做……"或"具有做……的能力"时，为可数名词。例如：He has a great academic ability.（他很有学术才能。）本例中 ability 的用法属于后者，所以需要在前面加不定冠词 a。

正：HPV-positive cervical cancer cells with a higher level of *Oct4* also had <u>a stronger colony-forming ability</u> than did HPV-negative cervical cancer cells.

译文：*Oct4* 表达水平更高的 HPV 阳性宫颈癌细胞比 HPV 阴性宫颈癌细胞具有<u>更强的克隆形成能力</u>。

七、连词误用

例 27 误：The research of depressive disorders is <u>not only</u> a major task currently,<u>but also</u> has far-reaching implications for medical development.

分析：关联词组 "not only...but also..." 强调递进关系的人或事物，可连接两个并列的谓语部分或句子，但不能分别接名词和谓语部分。

正：<u>Not only</u> is the research of depressive disorders a major task currently,<u>but</u> it <u>also</u> has far-reaching implications for medical development.

译文：当前，对抑郁症的研究<u>不仅</u>是一项重大任务，<u>而且</u>对于医疗发展有着重要的影响。

例 28 误：<u>Because</u> the existence of predicted miRNAs has yet to be validated, no accurate miRNA sequence could be used to synthesize accurate primer.

分析：本例中"被预测的 miRNA 是否存在有待进一步证实"是背景而不是原因，因此不能用 because 来引导。given that 意为"鉴于，考虑到"，表示基于某背景，用在此处更为合适。

正：<u>Given that</u> the existence of predicted miRNAs has yet to be validated, no accurate miRNA sequence could be used to synthesize accurate primers.

译文：<u>由于</u>被预测的 miRNA 是否存在尚未得到证实，<u>因此</u>，没有 miRNA 的精确序列可以用来合成精确的引物。

八、介词误用

1. 介词选用有误

例 29 误：Many other patients with Alzheimer's have <u>with</u> all probability inherited one or more of a group of about seven genes that increase the tendency to develop its symptoms.

分析：probability 意为"可能性，概率"，"很有可能"可以表述成 in all probability，with 不能与 probability 搭配。

正：Many other patients with Alzheimer's have <u>in</u> all probability inherited one or more of a group of about seven genes that increase the tendency to develop its symptoms.

译文：很多其他患阿尔茨海默病的患者都非常有可能因遗传得到了大约 7 个基因构成的一组基因中的 1 个或多个，从而增加了他们患该综合征的可能性。

例 30 误：We evaluated the effect of preoperative left ventricular function <u>to</u> early and late prognoses in 103 patients with aortic stenosis.

分析：effect 为名词，意为"效应，影响，结果"，在表达"对……的影响"时，后面常跟介词 on。常见固定表达 have an effect on sth. "对……产生影响"。本句中介词应改为 the effect of A on B。

正：We evaluated the effect of preoperative left ventricular function <u>on</u> early and late prognoses in 103 patients with aortic stenosis.

译文：我们对 103 例主动脉狭窄患者术前左室功能对早期和晚期预后的影响做了评价。

例 31 误：However, the decrease in MSNA was correlated to the decrease <u>of</u> right atrial pressure.

分析：decrease 意为"减少，降低"，若与 of 搭配表示"减少（某幅度）"，后面通常跟数字，如 a decrease of 5%；与 in 搭配表示"在……方面减少"，通常跟某个方面，如 The island gradually decreases in size.（这个小岛在逐渐缩小。）

正：However, the decrease in MSNA was correlated to the decrease <u>in</u> right atrial pressure.

译文：然而，MSNA 的降低与右心房压力降低有关。

例 32 误:In this study, pancolonic dye spraying was utilised to aid the detection of mucosal irregularities, instead of the categorisation of such lesions once found.

分析:instead of 意为"代替,作为……的替换"。例如:Now I can walk to work instead of going by car.(现在我可以步行去上班,而不必开车了。)as opposed to 意为"而,相对于",表示对比。例如:Two hundred people attended the meeting, as opposed to 300 the previous year.(今年有200人参加了会议,而去年是 300 人。)句中表达强调对比关系,因此应该使用 as opposed to。

正:In this study, pancolonic dye spraying was utilised to aid the detection of mucosal irregularities, as opposed to the categorisation of such lesions once found.

译文:本研究中,全结肠染色是用来帮助检测黏膜的异常,而不是对发现的异常病灶进行分类。

2. 介词和名词搭配有误

例 33 误:Certain medicines increase sensitivity for the sun.

分析:sensitivity 作"敏感性,过敏性"讲时,后面一般接介词 to,表示"对……的敏感性"。

正:Certain medicines increase sensitivity to the sun.

译文:某些药物会增加对阳光的敏感度。

例 34 误:There was no difference about the expression of *DNMT1* and *DNMT3B* among these three cell lines.

分析:本句中 difference 意为"差别,差异"。若表达"在……存在差异"后面常跟的介词是 in.

正:There was no difference in the expression of *DNMT1* and *DNMT3B* among these three cell lines.

译文:这三种宫颈癌细胞株之间无 *DNMT1* 和 *DNMT3B* 表达的差异。

例 35 误:BCL11A emerges as a therapeutic target of reactivation of HbF in beta-hemoglobin disorders.

分析:"作为治疗……的靶点"可以表达成"the target for..."。

正:BCL11A emerges as a therapeutic target for reactivation of HbF in beta-hemoglobin disorders.

译文:BCL11A 可以在 β-血红蛋白障碍性疾病中作为一个 HbF 重新激活的治疗靶点。

例 36 误:Considerable research for normal and diseased states within the retina has focused on neurons.

分析:表达"对……的研究",research 后应该接介词 on,而不是 for。

正:Considerable research on normal and diseased states within the retina has focused on neurons.

译文:大量对正常和病变的视网膜的研究工作集中于神经元。

(刘晓燕)

第二章　语　法

语法是语言的基石,要撰写出一篇优秀的英文学术论文,作者必须具备扎实的英语语法基础。由于汉语和英语在语法体系上存在巨大差异,受汉语语法思维定势的影响,中国作者撰写的英文学术论文中经常会出现一些语法错误。其中,出现频率较高的有下面几种:一致性原则错误、时态错误、语态错误等。下面介绍英文学术论文写作中经常涉及的一些语法知识。

第一节　一致性原则

英语要求在句子的构成中,不同的组成单元之间要一致,也就是一致性原则(the rule of agreement)。要保持一致的因素有很多,英文学术论文写作中经常会出现问题而特别需要注意的有:主语和谓语要一致;修饰语与主语名词要一致;代词和其代替的先行项要一致。

一、主语和谓语

主谓一致包括两种情况:主谓单复数一致和主谓逻辑关系一致。

1. 主语和谓语单复数　和汉语不同,英语中名词有单数和复数形式,动词也有单数和复数形式。主语和谓语的单复数要一致。中国作者不太习惯英语的这一语法规则,很难做到不假思索地配对,需要特别留心才能不出错误,特别是当主语名词中心词和动词分开时,更容易出错。

例 1　误:A series of processes precede the observed condition.

分析:这句话的主语是 a series,而不是 processes,主语是单数,因此后面的谓语动词 precede 也用单数。

正:A series of processes precedes the observed condition.

例 2　误:The Child Oral Health Related Quality of Life(COHRQOL)of three groups of children aged 12–15 years were surveyed with Child Oral Health Impact Profile(COHIP)(儿童口腔健康影响概况)。

分析:句子的主语中心词是 COHRQOL,而不是邻近的 years,所以谓语动词应该是单数形式的 was。

正:The Child Oral Health Related Quality of Life(COHRQOL)of three groups of children aged 12–15 years was surveyed with Child Oral Health Impact Profile(COHIP)。

下面几种特殊情况需要特别注意：

（1）以 -s 结尾的疾病名称。英语中有一些疾病名称是以 -s 结尾的，如 arthritis（关节炎）、bronchitis（支气管炎）、rickets（软骨病）、mumps（腮腺炎）、diabetes（糖尿病）、phlebitis（静脉炎）等，这类名词通常作单数用，谓语动词也应该用单数。例如：

Mumps is a kind of infectious disease.

Arthritis is a disease causing pain and swelling in the joints of the body.

但也有一些疾病名称既可作单数也可作复数用。例如：

Generally measles（麻疹）occurs in children.

Measles are sometimes caused by a tapeworm（绦虫）.

Rickets is/are caused by malnutrition（营养不良）.

（2）学术论文中经常出现的一些集合名词，如：class、team、group 等，既可作单数，也可作复数。若将该名词所表示的集体视为一个整体，动词用单数；若将侧重点放在组成集体的成员上，动词用复数。试比较下面两个句子：

The control group were given the same amount of sterile saline as in the rhES group for 14 days.

That group of subjects belongs to the upper social class.

（3）英语中描写质量、体积、时间（如：g、mg、l、ml、hour、second）等的词作主语时，谓语动词往往用单数。例如：

2 g was reduced.

3 ml was added.

7 hours was the required incubation time.

但如果是表示分次添加或减少时，谓语动词用复数。

7 ml were added stepwise（逐步地）.

（4）一些学术论文中常见的英语单词，如 datum、criterion、phenomenon、medium、stratum 的复数形式不规则，它们的复数形式分别是 data、criteria、phenomena、media、strata。例如：

The phenomena were not fully explained in those data.

2. 主语和谓语逻辑关系　语言根植于文化，中西方文化和思维习惯的差异导致中文和英文的表达方式有所不同。英语作为一种外语，其学习过程势必会受到汉语的干扰，最明显地体现在汉语意念的简单英语化（即字面上的生硬转化），导致英文中主语和谓语逻辑关系不一致。中文常说的一句话"你的身体很健康"，很多人可能会翻译成 your body is very healthy，但在地道的英文中，body 不能做 be healthy 的主语，它的主语应该是人。因此，这句中文应该翻译为 you are in good/excellent health。在写英文学术论文时要注意辨别谓语动词的真正主语。

例 3　误：The order of their morbidity（发病率）from high to low was the elbow, the shoulder, and the hip joints in turn.

分析：句子的主干是 the order was the elbow, the shoulder, and the hip joints。显然主谓逻

辑关系不一致。

正：The morbidity was in the following decreasing order：the elbow，the shoulder，the hip joints.

例 4 误：The control group except without performing moxibustion（艾灸），and other conditions were all the same with the experimental group.

分析：句子主语 other conditions 和谓语中的 the experimental group 不是同类事物，无法形成比较关系。因此，主语应改为 the treatments，谓语中加上 those for，这样主语和谓语在逻辑上才能保持一致。

正：The treatments for the control group were all the same as（those）for the experimental group except for moxibustion.

例 5 误：Therefore，it is reasonable to hypothesize that an abnormal SBP recovery ratio（卧位血压恢复率）appears to be due to exercise-induced impairment of left ventricular function（心室功能）.

分析：句子中的 that 宾语从句是从中文到英文的字面上的生硬转化，主语 an abnormal SBP recovery ratio 和其后面的谓语 appears to be due to... 逻辑关系上不一致。

正：Therefore，it is reasonable to hypothesize that the appearance of an abnormal SBP recovery ratio is due to exercise-induced impairment of left ventricular function.

写英文学术论文时，为了避免主语和谓语在逻辑上不一致，首先要熟悉英语的基本语法、词汇和文化背景；其次，要认识到中英文的差异，切忌信手拈来按字面硬译。将汉语句子翻译成英语，最基础的任务就是完全领会中文原意，然后通过对这些基本意义元素进行修饰，将其转换为地道的英文，也就是英语句子要表达的意义，最后再用适当的字词按照一定的语法规则进行变化后连缀成句。

二、修饰语和主语名词

英文学术论文写作中，充当修饰语的主要有动名词（gerund）、分词短语（participle phrase）和不定式短语（infinitive）。此时修饰语中的动词与主句的主语名词关系上要一致，即修饰语的逻辑主语应该就是主句的主语。这种句型结构相对复杂，且此类错误不容易被人察觉，因而在学术论文中出错的概率较高。

1. 动名词作修饰语

例 6 误：After finishing the purification，the activity of the isolated compound（分离化合物）was then studied.

分析：动名词 finishing the purification 的逻辑主语应该是人，而不是主句中的主语 the activity of the isolated compound，因此例句中修饰语和主语名词关系上不一致。

正：After finishing the purification，we studied the activity of the isolated compound.

例 7 误：After reviewing the X-rays，the patient had a lung operation.

分析：动名词 reviewing the X-rays 的逻辑主语应是医生，而不是患者。

正：After <u>the surgeon</u> reviewed the X-rays，the patient had a lung operation.

或：After <u>the X-rays</u> were reviewed，the patient had a lung operation.

2. 分词短语做修饰语

例 8 误：<u>Six woody plants</u> were investigated in this research，<u>aiming at</u> finding out some species that can be widely used in phytoremediation（植物修复）to deal with heavy metals in soil.

分析：aiming at 和主句主语 six woody plants 在关系上不一致，它的逻辑主语应该是 this research 或者 we。

正：<u>This research</u> investigated six woody plants，aiming at finding out some species that can be widely used in phytoremediation to deal with heavy metals in soil.

3. 不定式短语作修饰语

例 9 误：<u>To determine</u> the cause of delayed ductal closure（导管封闭）in fetal lambs（胎羊）that have experimental pulmonic stenosis（肺动脉狭窄），<u>pulmonic stenosis</u> was induced in fetal lambs at ages 70–77 days.

分析：动词不定式 To determine... 的逻辑主语应是 we，而不是 pulmonic stenosis。

正：To determine the cause of delayed ductal closure in fetal lambs that have experimental pulmonic stenosis，<u>we</u> induced pulmonic stenosis in fetal lambs at ages 70–77 days.

例 10 误：<u>To test</u> this hypothesis，<u>the *FGFR2* gene</u> in two strains of mice was disrupted（破坏）.

分析：不定式 To test... 的逻辑主语应是 we，而不是主句主语 the *FGFR2* gene。

正：To test this hypothesis，<u>we</u> disrupted the *FGFR2* gene in two strains of mice.

三、代词和先行项

代词是代替名词的一种词类。代词和其代替的先行项要在数（单数或复数）、性（阴性或阳性）和人称上保持一致。

<u>Many related compounds</u> were synthesized（合成）and <u>their</u> antivirus activities were studied.

There was no significant difference in the rate of death between <u>patients with shock</u> who were treated with dopamine（多巴胺）as the first-line vasopressor agent（一线血管加压剂）and <u>those</u> who were treated with norepinephrine（去甲肾上腺素）.

上面两个例子分别使用形容词性物主代词 their 和复数指示代词 those 来代替前面的先行项 many related compounds 和 patients with shock。

用代词时，除了要保持数、性一致外，还要避免指代不清的情况出现，以免无法分辨指代内容而引起误解。

例 11 误：In addition，in recent years，<u>the rising frequency of food safety scandals</u> has provoked consumers' vigilance on food safety though <u>it</u> is unrelated to GM technology（转基因技术）.

分析：在句子中，人称代词 it 既可以理解为 the rising frequency of food safety scandals，也可以理解为 consumers' vigilance on food safety，指代不清，容易让读者产生误解。

正：In addition，in recent years，the rising frequency of food safety scandals has provoked consumers' vigilance on food safety though <u>these scandals</u> are unrelated to GM technology.

以下两点可以有效避免代词和其代替的先行项不一致:①代词尽量靠近其代替的先行项;②如果使用代词可能引起歧义,应该放弃使用代词,而是重复使用先行项名词或名词词组。

(姚秋慧)

第二节　时态的使用

时态是英语语法中的一个重要概念,表示行为发生的时间和说话时的关系,分为过去时、现在时和将来时。学术论文中的动词时态主要有现在时和过去时(偶尔也会出现将来时)。Day 曾详细指出学术论文中动词时态的使用原则:众所周知的事实(以往的研究结果)应使用现在时;方法和结果的描述应使用过去时;陈述部分应使用现在时,例如:Table one shows that...;责任的转移应使用过去时,例如:Hyland demonstrated that...。

一篇英文学术论文通常由以下五个部分组成:摘要(abstract)、引言(introduction)、材料和方法(materials and methods)、结果(results)和讨论(discussion)。下面分别论述这五个部分中时态的使用情况。

一、摘要

摘要中,过去时和现在时并用,以过去时为主。学术论文的摘要主要介绍研究的背景、目的、方法、结果和结论。研究的背景和结论多是陈述性的内容或从具体结果演绎出的一般性原理,一般用现在时;而研究的目的、方法和结果尚未得到承认,并且是写论文以前做的事情,一般用过去时。

例 1　This study <u>describes</u> development and validation of a questionnaire as an adjunct to traditional Chinese medicine diagnosis of Yin-Deficiency Syndrome(Yin-DS). The Yin-Deficiency Questionnaire 1(Yin-DQ1)<u>consists</u> of 10 items.(研究内容,用现在时)Seventy-nine healthy volunteers and 44 patients diagnosed with Yin-DS <u>were enrolled</u> for the evaluation of discriminant validity and factorial validity. Another group of 83 healthy volunteers <u>participated</u> for test-retest reliability test. Internal consistency <u>was</u> high in both groups(Cronbach's α=0.861 5). Test-retest reliability(Spearman's rank correlation coefficient)<u>ranged</u> from 0.54 to 0.79(P <0.01). Factor analysis <u>demonstrated</u> that a two-factor solution best <u>explained</u> the variance in responses(51.62%). The scores of all items in patients diagnosed with Yin-DS <u>were</u> significantly higher compared with those of healthy volunteers. The data <u>showed</u> the internal consistency,test-retest reliability and strong discriminative properties of the Yin-DQ1.(研究过程和结果,用过去时)

例 2　Large-scale natural disasters,such as earthquakes,tsunamis,volcanic eruptions,and typhoons,<u>occur</u> worldwide.(研究背景,用现在时)After the Great East Japan earthquake and tsunami, our medical support operation's experiences <u>suggested</u> that traditional medicine might be useful for treating the various symptoms of the survivors. (过去的事情,用过去时) However, little information <u>is</u> available regarding herbal medicine treatment in such situations. (研究背景,用现在时) Considering that further disasters will occur, we <u>performed</u> a literature review and <u>summarized</u> the traditional medicine approaches for treatment after large-scale disasters. We <u>searched</u> PubMed and Cochrane Library for articles written in English, and Ichushi for those written in Japanese. Articles published before 31 March 2016 <u>were</u> included. Keywords "disaster" and "herbal medicine" <u>were</u> used in our search. Among studies involving herbal medicine after a disaster, we <u>found</u> two randomized controlled trials investigating post-traumatic stress disorder (PTSD), three retrospective investigations of trauma or common diseases, and seven case series or case reports of dizziness, pain, and psychosomatic symptoms. (研究过程和结果,用过去时) In conclusion, herbal medicine <u>has been</u> used to treat trauma, PTSD, and other symptoms after disasters. However, few articles <u>have been</u> published, likely due to the difficulty in designing high quality studies in such situations. Further study <u>is needed</u> to clarify the usefulness of herbal medicine after disasters. (研究结论,用现在时)

二、引言

引言主要使用现在时。引言是论文正文的第一部分,为读者提供理解论文及其重要性的必要背景知识,指明研究的主要问题和理论依据,并阐明研究目的。引言的基本时态是现在时,因为本部分主要表述相关领域的研究现状(已发表的成果视为事实)。

例 3 Traditional Chinese medicine (TCM) <u>has made</u> great contributions by maintaining the health and treating the diseases of the Chinese people for thousands of years (Tong *et al.*, 2012a; Li *et al.*, 2014; Wang *et al.*, 2014a; Hao and Jiang, 2015). However, there <u>are issues</u> in the development of TCM, with one of the most important tasks being to improve treatment efficacy by using the adequate herbal medicine dosage (Xu, 2005; Xu *et al.*, 2013). The clinical therapeutics of TCM <u>constitutes</u> a complicated process "theory-methodology-formulation-medication-dosage", in which a formula prescription with a specific herbal dosage <u>is</u> particularly essential (Tang *et al.*, 2008, 2012; Fu *et al.*, 2013a). Clearly, after the correct diagnosis and formula prescription, selecting accurate dosages of each herbal drug in the formulation <u>is</u> the key to ensuring the clinical efficacy and safety. Thus, a full understanding of the precise herbal dose selection <u>has</u> a critical importance in the daily TCM practice to deliver the best treatment to patients suffering from different diseases (Tong *et al.*, 2012b; Xiao *et al.*, 2015). (研究现状,用现在时)

例 4 In the last few years, the importance of regulatory small RNAs (核糖核酸) as mediators of a number of cellular processes in bacteria <u>has begun</u> to be recognized. (研究背景,时间标志词 the last few years,用现在完成时,表示过去的事情对现在的影响) Although instances of naturally occurring antisense RNAs <u>have been known</u> for many years, the participation of sRNAs in protein tagging for degradation, modulation of RNA polymerase（聚合酶）activity, and stimulation of translation <u>are</u> relatively recent discoveries（for review, see Wassarman *et al.*, 1999; Wassarman and Storz, 2000）. These findings <u>have raised</u> questions about how extensively sRNAs <u>are</u> used, what other cellular activities <u>might be</u> regulated by sRNAs, and what other mechanisms of action <u>exist</u> for sRNAs. In addition, prokaryotic（原核的）sRNAs <u>appear</u> to target different cellular functions than their eukaryotic（真核的）counterparts that primarily <u>act</u> during RNA biogenesis. It <u>is</u> unclear whether this apparent difference between prokaryotic and eukaryotic sRNAs <u>is</u> accurate or <u>stems</u> from the incompleteness of current knowledge. Implicit in these questions <u>is</u> the question of how many sRNAs <u>exist</u> in a given organism and whether the current known sRNAs <u>are</u> truly representative of sRNA function in general.（研究现状，用现在时）

通常情况下，描述已发表的文献成果时应该用现在时。但如果文献的作者作为主语，根据 Day 的英文学术论文中的时态使用原则，为了转移责任，通常使用过去时。

请比较下面两个句子。

Greenberg <u>showed</u> that streptomycin inhibited *S. nocolor*.

Investigation by Greenberg <u>shows</u> that streptomycin inhibits *S. nocolor*.

三、材料和方法

材料和方法一般用过去时。本部分主要描述具体的实验和数据分析过程，包括使用的材料、工具、方法等。因为这部分内容是在写文章之前做的事情，并且还没被接受为事实，因此一般用过去时。

例 5 Selection of TCM+and TCM-Samples

TCM+samples <u>were selected</u> from the published well-known TCM prescriptions.（实验过程，用过去时）As the majority of TCM prescriptions <u>contain</u> four to ten constituent herbs（客观事实，用现在时）, those with less or more numbers of herbs <u>were not considered</u> in this work. These prescriptions <u>were screened</u> to remove those with incomplete information about the traditionally defined properties of their constituent herbs. A total of 647 well-known TCM prescriptions <u>were selected</u> from this process, which <u>were randomly divided</u> into a training set of 575 prescriptions and an independent testing set of 72 prescriptions for training and testing our SVM classification system.（实验过程，用过去时）The list of these prescriptions and their distribution into the training/testing sets <u>are given</u> in Appendixes 1 to 7.（客观陈述，用现在时）

例 6 Development of Yin-DQ1

Yin-Deficiency Questionnaire 1（Yin-DQ1）<u>was developed</u> as a first step for developing and validating a set of adjunctive diagnostic tools in TCM. Based on the literature search of symptoms of Yin-DS（Yang, 1995）, the preliminary Yin-DQ with 12 items <u>was designed and checked</u> for content validity by three Korean medicine doctors（KMDs）with more than 5 years of clinical experience. It <u>was pre-tested</u> in a group of college students in Korea and taken together with advice from other KMDs and statisticians to check for face validity. Through this process, the complete Yin-DQ1 <u>was developed</u>. (实验过程,用过去时)The Yin-DQ1 <u>consists</u> of 10 items of symptoms, each scored by the patient on a 100 mm Visual Analog Scale (VAS), from 0 (never) to 10 (almost all the time). (客观陈述,用现在时)The questionnaire <u>was administered</u> face to face and <u>supposed</u> to be checked based on the patient's last six months' experience. (实验过程,用过去时)The higher score <u>implicates</u> more frequent symptom manifestation. (客观陈述,用现在时)The items <u>are</u> as follows: (客观陈述,用现在时)for primary symptoms of Yin-DS, the examiners <u>assessed</u> irritable fever on the five Hearts (the heart, two palms, and two soles), flushing of the zygomatic (颧) area in the afternoon, tidal fever, and night sweating. For secondary symptoms of Yin-DS, the questionnaire <u>assessed</u> emaciation or weight loss, dried mouth and/or throat, dizziness, insomnia, decreased amount of urine with yellowish color and constipation (Appendix 1). Two items "reddened tongue with little coating" and "minute and frequent pulse" of tongue and pulse diagnoses <u>were excluded</u> after pre-test because these parameters could be prone to measuring errors. It <u>took</u> an average of 5 min to fill out the Yin-DQ1, showing a low respondent-burden. (实验过程,用过去时)

Validity Testing

Validity <u>is</u> concerned with the accuracy of data, that is, ensuring responses <u>are</u> a true reflection of the issues of interest (Smith, 2002). (引用已发表的文献,用现在时)To test construct validity, both the factorial validity and discriminant validity <u>had to</u> be determined. Seventy-nine healthy college students and office workers <u>volunteered and comprised</u> the control group. Forty-four outpatients diagnosed with Yin-DS by a KMD at the Kyung Hee University Medical Center in Seoul, Korea, from September to October 2003, <u>were allocated</u> to the Yin-DS group (Group A, n=123). The three KMDs who <u>made</u> diagnoses <u>had</u> more than 5 years of clinical experience in the kidney and endocrine (内分泌) unit of Kyung Hee University Medical Center and the patients <u>were diagnosed</u> as Yin-DS by one of the three KMDs and <u>prescribed</u> herbal formula for their conditions no more than one month prior to this study. Participants <u>were asked</u> to complete the Yin-DQ1, and the scores for each item were analyzed. (实验过程,用过去时)

Statistical Analysis

Data analyses <u>were performed</u> using SPSS version 11.0 (SPSS Inc., USA). Data <u>are presented</u> as mean ± SD unless stated otherwise. (客观陈述,用现在时)Internal consistency of the Yin-DQ1 <u>was examined</u> by computing item-total correlations and Cronbach's α. To test construct validity, both factorial validity and discriminant validity <u>were evaluated</u>: factor analysis <u>was performed</u> using principal component extraction and variance maximizing (varimax) rotation with an Eigen value over 1.5 as the criteria; discriminant validity <u>was assessed</u> using the student's t-test in group A. (实验数据分析,用过去时)

四、结果

结果通常使用过去时。本部分展示材料和方法中所述的实验得出的主要结果。同材料和方法一样,这部分的内容还没被接受为事实,基本时态仍为过去时。

例7　Internal Consistency

Cronbach's α <u>was</u> 0.861 5 for the mean of the item-total and <u>did not change</u> significantly on removing of any of the 10 items. Each item <u>had</u> an item-total correlation value greater than 0.5 and two items (flushing of the zygomatic area in the afternoon and tidal fever) <u>had</u> correlation values greater than 0.6 (Table 2). (数据分析结果,用过去时)

Factor Analysis

The 10 items <u>were subjected</u> to factor analysis to examine the factorial validity of the Yin-DQ1 using principal component extraction and varimax rotation with an Eigen value over 1.5 as the criteria. The two-factor solution <u>made</u> the most conceptual sense and <u>explained</u> an acceptable amount of variance (50.62%) in the response (Table 4). Factor 1 (Deficient-Heat Symptoms) <u>was made</u> up of 4 items with factor loadings of 0.539 to 0.819, which <u>explained</u> 25.97% of variance. These 4 items <u>included</u>: irritable fever on the five Hearts, flushing of the zygomatic area in the afternoon, tidal fever, and dried mouth and/or throat. Factor 2 (Accompanying Symptoms) <u>consisted</u> of remaining 6 items of night sweats, emaciation, dizziness, insomnia, decreased amount of urine with yellowish color, and constipation. It explained 24.65% of the variance. (实验结果,用过去时)

Discriminant Validity

Discriminant validity <u>was assessed</u> by comparing the mean difference of scores on each item between the Yin-DS group and the control group (student's *t*-test). The two groups <u>showed</u> significant difference on every item (Table 5). (实验结果,用过去时)

例8　Younger patients <u>had</u> a worse disease free survival (greater probability of recurrence) at all time periods (Figure 1; $P<0.001$). In 5 years, the actuarial recurrence rate for patients<35 years old <u>was</u> 30.4% as compared with 18.7% for older patients. This difference <u>persisted</u> in 10 years, at which time the actuarial recurrence rates (精算复发率) <u>were</u> 40.1% and 28.6% respectively. Overall survival among young patients <u>was</u> significantly worse than that for older patients (Figure 1; $P=0.002$). The 5-year survival rate <u>was</u> 80% for patients aged<35 years as compared with 88.5% for older patients. (数据分析结果,用过去时)

以下这种情况需要注意:

陈述表格(table)或图表(figure)呈现的结果时,一般用现在时。

Figure 2 <u>shows</u> the percentage of districts in Washington, D. C. that have individuals identified as filling particular primary positions.

The characteristics of cases and controls <u>are</u> shown in Table 1. (Table 1 shows the characteristics of cases and controls.)

五、讨论

讨论中各种时态交替使用。讨论是在评论研究过程和研究结果的基础上,将研究个体问题得出的结论放到一个更大的领域中考量,得出具有推广借鉴意义的结论,体现研究的价值。本部分的动词时态相对复杂,根据语言信息的不同,过去时、现在时和将来时可能会交替使用。同时,本部分经常使用情态动词,使结论和观点更为客观。

例9 We developed and validated a questionnaire to help objective diagnosis of Yin-DS in TCM. The newly developed Yin-DQ1 was found to be reliable and valid. The items demonstrated good internal consistency and test-retest reliability was excellent for all items. The two-factor solution explained an acceptable level of variance and the questionnaire showed strong discriminant properties.(总结研究过程和结果,用过去时)Given these findings, the Yin-DQ1 can be considered a good adjunct(辅助手段)to help diagnose Yin-DS in a more objective manner.(研究结论,用现在时)

Reliability is concerned with the repeatability or reproducibility of measurement(Smith,2002).(引用已发表的文献,用现在时)To test reliability, the authors evaluated internal consistency and test-retest reliability.(实验过程,用过去时)Cronbach's α measures how well a set of items or variables measures a single unidimensional latent construct. Its value ranges from 0 to 1 and the higher the score, the more reliable the generated scale is.(客观陈述,用现在时)It has been indicated that 0.7 is an acceptable reliability coefficient, but lower thresholds are sometimes used in the literature(Nunnaly,1978).(引用已发表的文献,用现在时)Cronbach's α coefficient for the Yin-DQ1 showed strong internal consistency(研究结果,用过去时),with a value of 0.8615 and therefore, it may be considered to be a reliable measurement of Yin-DS(研究结论,用现在时). In test-retest reliability, Spearman's rank correlation coefficients demonstrated that the strength of association was highly significant for all items(研究结果,用过去时)and the Yin-DQ1 is considered stable between administrations(研究结论,用现在时).

...

There are limitations and future research questions to be tested in the Yin-DQ1. First, the Yin-DQ1 may not be sufficient to replace the individualized differential TCM diagnosis by an experienced practitioner. It should be stressed that the Yin-DQ1 was originally developed as a reliable adjunctive instrument of TCM diagnosis which could otherwise be arbitrary(since it is based on the assessment of individual practitioners). As it is devoid of the items on tongue and pulse diagnoses which may be regarded as important in TCM diagnosis, caution should be taken to identify whether(1)the results of the questionnaire are in accordance with the assessments of the experienced practitioners and(2)they agree especially with the tongue and pulse diagnoses.(研究的局限性,用现在时)

Nevertheless, the findings of this study suodot that Yin-DQ1 serves as an adjunctive diagnostic tool, and further research is needed to determine its responsiveness to longitudinal changes to be used as a visualized method to assess the degree of Yin-DS in a clinical trial.（研究结论，用现在时）

例 10　These results indicate that cancer genome sequencing of large collections of samples will yield new insights into cancer not anticipated by existing knowledge.（研究结论，用现在时和将来时）

时态的用法没有严格的规定。现在越来越多的作者除了实验部分用过去时，其他部分都用现在时。美国化学会的 *ACA Style Guide* 建议实验部分用过去时，其他部分可以用过去时，也可以用现在时，但要保持一致。

（姚秋慧）

第三节　语态的使用

语态（voice）作为一个语法范畴，是表示主语和动词之间的主动或被动关系的动词形式。英语动词有两种语态：主动语态（active voice）和被动语态（passive voice）。当主语为动作执行者即施动者时，动词用主动语态；如果主语是动作的承受者即受动者，动词用被动语态。因此，在强调动作的承受者或动作的执行者无法确定、不重要或难以说出时，可以用被动语态。

比较下面两个句子：

Researchers at the University of California discovered a new genetic link to diabetes（糖尿病）.

A new genetic link to diabetes was discovered by researchers at the University of California.

和主动句相比，被动句中的主语 A new genetic link to diabetes 得到特别强调。

被动语态不提及动作的执行者，排除主观成分，比主观语态显得更客观，因此在英文学术论文的写作中大量应用。然而，国外科学写作界从 20 世纪 60—70 年代开始摒弃被动语态的文风，不少科学写作组织（如美国医学会）、编辑组织（如《科学》杂志）明确主张使用主动语态，以使科学论文和著作的文字生动、有活力、语言简洁明确；多用人称代词 we，增强作者的责任感和对工作客观描述的亲切感、生动性。

比较下面两个句子：

In 2002, it was reported by the authors of this paper that the synthesis of anthramycin analogues（合成的安定霉素类似物）and their DNA binding activities was studied by gel electrophoresis（凝胶电泳）.

In 2002, we reported that the synthesis of anthramycin analogues and their DNA binding activities was studied by gel electrophoresis.

显然，把 it was reported by the authors of this paper that 改为 we reported that 显得更简要，

更直接。

英文学术论文中还经常使用以下句型来增强作者的责任感：

This paper reports...

The writer concludes...

We made the analysis...

The researchers have carried out...

虽然提倡在英文学术论文写作中更多地使用主动语态，但是依然可以使用被动语态。在描述现象和实验过程时，主要使用被动语态。

These cellular components <u>have been called</u> the "genealogy-defining core", the "genetic core" of cells or the "functional core of genomes", and their common history <u>has been cited</u> as the strongest support for the three-domain tree.

Validity <u>is concerned</u> with the accuracy of data, that is, ensuring responses are a true reflection of the issues of interest (Smith, 2002). To test construct validity, both the factorial validity and discriminant validity <u>had to be determined</u>. Seventy-nine healthy college students and office workers volunteered and comprised the control group. Forty-four outpatients diagnosed with Yin-DS by a KMD at the Kyung Hee University Medical Center in Seoul, Korea, from September to October 2003, <u>were allocated</u> to the Yin-DS group (Group A, $n=123$). The three KMDs who made diagnoses had more than 5 years of clinical experience in the kidney and endocrine unit of Kyung Hee University Medical Center and the patients <u>were diagnosed</u> as Yin-DS by one of the three KMDs and <u>prescribed</u> herbal formula for their conditions no more than one month prior to this study. Participants <u>were asked</u> to complete the Yin-DQ1, and the scores for each item were analyzed.

练习

1. 请为下列句子选择正确的动词形式。

（1）Two aftershocks of the heart attack [was, were] almost as serious as the original attack itself.

（2）Phlebitis [is, are] a swollen condition of the blood vessels.

（3）The audience [was, were] very responsive to her appeal for aid.

（4）5 g [was, were] reduced stepwise.

（5）2 hours [is, are] needed to finish the questionnaire.

（6）In contrast, the nuclei of apoptotic cells [was, were] stained yellow and brown.

（7）Neither the general nor his men [was, were] prepared for the bitterly cold winter; not only the men but their leader [was, were] ready to retreat.

（8）Free market enterprise or socialism [is, are] the direction of the future.

2. 请修改下列句子。

（1）The expression of *Oct4* in both Hela and Caski cells was also higher than C-33A cells.

（2）Methodological comparison shows that the SPR biosensor has the same detection rate as traditional culture methods（$P<0.05$）.

（3）To determine functional role of YB1 in prostate cancer cell invasion，YB1 gene expression in PC3 cells was silenced.

（4）Hyland demonstrated that cervical cancers contained a subpopulation of stem-like cancer cells expressing Oct4 protein.

（5）The abnormal expression of miRNAs may involve in human diseases，including cancer.

（6）In traditional Chinese medicine theory，Zheng，which was also called a syndrome or pattern，was the basic unit and a key concept.

（7）Figure 1 showed the amounts of pollution accumulated in China over the past two decades.

（8）The purpose of this article will be to give the most direct answer possible to the direct question of how long advertising affects sales.

3. 请找出下列段落中的错误并改正。

Music，meditation and acupuncture are used to relieve stress. For those who have developed a dependency on tranquilizers，it is most effective，as long as one could get used to the needles.

4. 请用适当的动词时态填空。

（1）Table 2 graphically _____（represent）the change in ecological footprint and biocapacity over this period. As can be seen，an ecological deficit _____（emerge）in 1991 and _____（increase）dramatically in subsequent years. Although both biocapacity and ecological footprint _____（grow）gradually，the increase in the ecological footprint（2.5 fold）_____（be）much greater than the corresponding biocapacity（1.4 fold）. In 2006，the ecological deficit _____（reach）1.05 gha，and the ecological footprint per capita _____（be）2.11 gha compared with the biocapacity per capita of 1.06 gha. The consistent increase in the ecological footprint _____（can）be directly related to population growth and economic development. The ecosystems _____（face）the twofold impact of population growth coupled with an increasing per capita consumption rate.

（2）Over the past three decades，many researchers and engineers _____（develop）several urban infrastructure designs to _____（meet）the dual needs of pavement stability and tree health. There _____ (be) two fundamental approaches to these designs: engineered soils and suspended pavement. Engineered soils _____ (be) composed of course stone _____ (mix) with fine-textured mineral soil to create a high porosity matrix that _____ (can) be compacted to engineering load-bearing standards yet _____ (retain) physical properties conducive to aeration, hydration, and root elongation.

5. 请用适当的动词语态填空。

TCM-samples _____ (generate) by randomly combining herbs into 4-, 5-, 6-, 7-, 8-, 9- and 10-herb recipes from a pool of 813 herbs with available information about their traditionally defined properties. These samples _____ (draw) in such a way that they _____ (distribute) evenly in the sampling space. They _____ (check) further to remove those that happen to be in the TCM+class. A total of 1,961 randomly assembled recipes _____ (select) from this process to form the TCM-training set. The number of samples in the 4-, 5-, 6-, 7-, 8-, 9- and 10-herb TCM-training set sub-groups are 501, 251, 211, 267, 231, 290 and 210, respectively. A total of 5,039 randomly assembled recipes _____ (use) as the TCM-testing set. The number of samples in the 4-, 5-, 6-, 7-, 8-, 9- and 10-herb TCM-testing set sub-groups are 499, 749, 789, 733, 769, 710 and 790, respectively.

（姚秋慧）

第三章 句 法

除了语法错误,中国作者在撰写英文学术论文中也会出现一些句法错误,如句子冗长重复、句子结构不完整、句式杂糅等。这些错误严重影响读者的阅读速度和理解程度,有时甚至会误导读者。为了避免句法错误的出现,需要掌握一些基本的英语句法知识。

第一节 句法基本知识

一、句子的类型

句子是语法结构的最高层次,也是构成语篇的基本语言单位。在英语中,句子可以分为两大类:简单句(simple sentence)和多重句(multiple sentence);多重句又包括并列句(compound sentence)、复合句(complex sentence)和并列复合句(compound-complex sentence)。

1. 简单句 简单句指只包括一个主谓结构的句子,简单句的各个成分都是由词或词组实现的。

例 1 Argumentation writing aims at convincing.

例 2 The major changes on consumer perception have occurred after 2010.

2. 并列句 并列句是由两个或两个以上的简单句并列连接而组成的句子。各个简单句彼此独立,互不依从,但表达的意思之间有一定关系。句子之间通常用并列连词连接。

例 3 The author has a point or a hypothesis, and he tries by all means to prove it.

例 4 The first sentence is the starting point of the entire text, so it introduces two keywords:liver transplantation and living donor.

3. 复合句 复合句由一个主句(main clause)和一个或多个从句(dependent clause)构成。主句是全句的主体;从句充当句子的某一成分,不能独立存在,须由一个关联词(connective)引导。根据在句中的作用,从句可以分为定语从句(attributive clause)、状语从句(adverbial clause)和名词性从句(noun clause)。名词性从句又包括主语从句(subject clause)、宾语从句(object clause)、表语从句(predicative clause)和同位语从句(appositive clause)。

例 5 The three patients who made diagnoses had more than 5 years of clinical experience.(定语从句)

例 6 We discovered that many of these small RNAs(核糖核酸)interact with the RNA-binding protein Hfq.(宾语从句)

例 7 Although there is mounting evidence that trees grow better and are healthier when planted in engineered soils rather than conventional tree pits, there is no empirical research, to our knowledge, that has investigated tree stability in engineered soils. (状语从句、同位语从句、定语从句)

4. 并列复合句 并列复合句同时具有并列句和复合句的特征。一个并列复合句包含两个或两个以上的主句,至少有一个主句又内含从句。

例 8 If the number of human miRNAs increases to 1,000, as recently predicted by Berezikov *et al.*, it will then be possible to profile miRNA expression using PCR; however, it may be less practical than microarrays.

例 9 When ship workers went on strike, several of their leaders were imprisoned, because union and the right to strike is not legal; however, domestic and international pressure forced the government to relent, although the unions remain weak by Western standards.

二、英文学术论文中的常见句式

受其学术性质的影响,学术论文的句式结构相对来说不是特别丰富。英文学术论文中比较常见的句式主要有:陈述句,祈使句,复合句,it 作形式主语的句式,as 引导的定语从句,表示比较的句式,含有 may、would 等情态动词表示推测的句式和含有 if、unless、given 等的条件句。

1. 陈述句 学术论文是在科学领域内表达科学研究成果的文章,主要陈述研究目的、内容、方法、结果和结论等。因而,英文学术论文中大部分是陈述句,而疑问句和感叹句使用很少。

例 10 There are two major advantages of TCM.

例 11 Systems biology can help to reveal the scientific connotation of TCM syndromes.

2. 祈使句 在描述实验过程或讨论实验结果时,论文中有时会使用祈使句。

例 12 Now let K equal to zero, and then we obtain the following equation.

例 13 Fill in the tube with cold water, and then heat the tube to 100℃ .

3. 复合句 复合句也是英文学术论文中的常见句型,用来表述研究中各种因素之间复杂的相互关系。

例 14 The clinical therapeutics of TCM constitutes a complicated process expressed as "theory-methodology-formulation-medication-dosage", in which a formula prescription with a specific herbal dosage is particularly essential.

例 15 In test-retest reliability, Spearman's rank correlation coefficients(相关系数) demonstrated that the strength of association was highly significant for all items and the Yin-DQ1 is considered stable between administrations.

4. It+be+*adj.*/participle+that clause 句式 为了保持句子的平衡和使所述内容显得更为客观,It+be+*adj.*/participle+that clause 句式在英文学术论文中比较常见。在此句式中,it 是形式主语,真正的主语是后面的 that 从句。

例 16 It has been indicated that 0.7 is an acceptable reliability coefficient, but lower thresholds are sometimes used in the literature.

例 17　<u>It should be stressed that</u> the Yin-DQ1 was originally developed as a reliable adjunctive instrument of TCM diagnosis which could otherwise be arbitrary（since it is based on the assessment of individual practitioners）.

5. as 引导的定语从句　英文学术论文中经常出现 as 引导的非限制性定语从句。在此句式中，as 表示主句的内容，意思为"正像""正如"。

例 18　<u>As is shown</u> in Table 2，each item had an item-total correlation value（相关值）greater than 0.5 and two items（flushing of the zygomatic area in the afternoon and tidal fever）had correlation values greater than 0.6.

例 19　<u>As is stated above</u>，the drug combination group and the chemotherapy group both had a flat growth curve.

6. 表示比较的句式　对照是学术研究实验设计的基本原则之一，因而学术论文中含有大量与比较相关的内容。英文学术论文中，表示比较的句式出现的频率也就比较高。例如：形容词或副词的比较级 +than、be similar to、the same as、differ（difference）between...and...、compared with 等。

例 20　The data suggest that the HEV（戊型肝炎病毒）could be <u>more widespread than</u> previously thought.

例 21　The scores of all items in patients diagnosed with Yin-DS <u>were significantly higher compared with</u> those of healthy volunteers.

例 22　One can argue that it is questionable to what extent the participants understood the questions and whether this understanding was <u>the same as</u> the clinicians administering the questionnaire.

例 23　In hospitalized patients，performance on Piagetian tasks of judgement <u>was similar to</u> that among children younger than 10 years of age.

7. 含有 may、would 等情态动词表示推测的句式　学术论文中的有些内容是作者的推测或假设，为了谨慎起见，作者常在英文学术论文中使用 may、would 等情态动词增强所述内容的客观性。

例 24　First，the Yin-DQ1 <u>may not be sufficient</u> to replace the individualized differential TCM diagnosis by an experienced practitioner.

例 25　It <u>would be necessary</u> later to investigate whether the Yin-DQ1 can distinguish Yin-DS patients and other non Yin-DS patients with similar symptoms.

8. 含有 if、unless、given 等的条件句　学术研究中的一些观点和假设只有在一定条件下才能成立，这时就需要用到条件句。

例 26　<u>If</u> adverse effects are thought to be associated with herbal medicines，treatment should be stopped，and a proper examination should be performed.

例 27　Data analyses were performed using SPSS version 11.0（SPSS Inc.，USA）. Data are presented as...<u>unless</u> stated otherwise.

三、句子的衔接

学术论文有很强的推理性。要表达一个思维过程,思想之间的传承和衔接要紧密、合理。思维是用句子表达出来的,这样句子之间的衔接和关系就特别重要。通过句子之间的衔接,作者就可以把前后的思想贯穿起来,从而达到说明、推理和讨论的目的。在英语中,句子之间的衔接可以通过连词(如:and、for、so、not only...but also...、neither...nor...、when、although、after、because、unless、although、where、whereas 等),具有衔接作用的副词(如:also、however、moreover、furthermore、therefore、otherwise、consequently、similarly、nevertheless、thus 等),介词(如:including、despite 等)和一些短语(如:as a result、in addition、in contrast、for example、in spite of 等)来实现。

根据所连接的句子之间的关系,英文学术论文中经常使用的衔接词和短语可以分为九类。

1. 因果关系 表示因果关系的词和短语有:as、because、since、so、therefore、consequently、thus、hence、as a result 等。

例 28 <u>As</u> it is devoid of the items on tongue and pulse diagnoses which may be regarded as important in TCM diagnosis, caution should be taken to identify whether ① the results of the questionnaire are in accordance with the assessments of the experienced practitioners and ② they agree especially with the tongue and pulse diagnoses.

例 29 <u>Because</u> the earth environments are complex, external and evaginated(外翻的) respiratory organs did not adapt to dry and changeful climate.

例 30 These are fundamental theories of traditional Chinese medicine, but they are entirely different from Western medicine. <u>So</u> many people think that traditional Chinese medicine is not a science.

2. 并列关系 当描述并列关系的事物或特性时,如果没有表示衔接的词或短语,往往给人留下罗列或前后关系不明的感觉。使用 furthermore、moreover、also、in addition、besides 等副词和短语可以使句子更通畅。

also、too 表示新陈述的内容与前面的同等重要,只是语气上有所不同。too 比较随便,日常用语中使用较多。also 要正式些,在英文学术论文中使用的最多。besides 引入的句子多用来补充和加强前面的句子。in addition、moreover 和 furthermore 多用于强调新引入的内容的重要性。

例 31 <u>In addition</u>, further testing is required to examine whether the Yin-DQ1 can be used in a clinical trial to test the efficacy of treatments for Yin-DS.

例 32 One common problem for both Western and traditional medicine is the insufficient transport of medicines. <u>Furthermore</u>, in disaster situations, clean drinking water, which is required to take some medicines, is often scarce.

例 33 Chlorins（绿素类）play important biological roles. They inhibit certain oxidative stress（氧化应激）in many marine species, including sponge, clam, and scallop. <u>Also</u>, one of the chlorins is a hormone（荷尔蒙）responsible for sexual development in a marine worm. <u>Moreover</u>, in addition to their natural functions, they showed potential applications in medical and material sciences.

3. 转折关系 表示转折关系的连词和副词有：but、yet、however、nevertheless、nonetheless 等。

例 34 Nausea, diarrhea, and malaise were observed with the use of XTJYF, <u>but</u> the symptoms were not considered serious, and there were no significant differences between the XTJYF and placebo groups.

例 35 Aspirin is recommended to prevent myocardial infarction（心肌梗死）and graft occlusion（移植物闭塞）. <u>However</u>, aspirin is also associated with bleeding.

4. 对比关系 表示对比关系的连词和短语有：in/by contrast、whereas、while 等。

例 36 In most cases, the conservation between *E. coli* and *Salmonella* was>85%, <u>whereas</u> that of the typical gene encoding an ORF was frequently<70%.

例 37 Angelicae Radix, Paeoniae Radix, and other herbs are thought to support blood production, <u>while</u> Rehmanniae Radix, Ophiopogonis Radix, and others reinforce liquid formation.

5. 相似关系 表示相似关系的连接词有：similarly、likewise 等。

例 38 Tonifying drugs（补药）enhance energy uptake through digestion and absorption（in the case of Panax ginseng Radix）or through respiration（in the case of Astragali Radix）. <u>Similarly</u>, Angelicae Radix, Paeoniae Radix, and other herbs are thought to support blood production, while Rehmanniae Radix, Ophiopogonis Radix, and others reinforce liquid formation.

6. 条件关系 对于前后相连的两个句子，当其中一个句子的成立以另一个为条件时，句子之间就需要用到表示条件关系的连接词，如 unless、if、given（that）等。

例 39 Data analyses were performed using SPSS version 11.0（SPSS Inc., USA）. Data are presented as mean ± SD <u>unless</u> stated otherwise（除非另有说明）.

例 40 In the present study, the term "challenge test" was used only <u>if</u> cautious readministration of Kampo medicine was conducted by a physician; liver injuries which reappeared upon voluntary retaking of causal medicine by patients and which were caused by unwitting readministration by physicians were excluded from this study.

7. 举例 学术论文中经常用举例的方法来细化或论证前面所述的内容，英文中通常使用 for example、for instance、specifically、such as、including 等词或词组来引出后面的例子。

例 41 The circadian rhythm（昼夜节律）of illness has been emphasized for thousands of years in traditional Chinese medicine（TCM）, using this knowledge to schedule therapies <u>such as</u> acupuncture during appropriate hours of the day.

例 42 In shelters, long-term evacuees complain of numerous health problems, <u>including</u> infectious disease, pain, insomnia, or chronic disease.

例 43 The population growth in the US is affected by many factors, <u>such as</u> race, religion, income, and cultures. For instance, Jewish family has an average birth rate of 3.4 children per couple and Caucasian white family has a birth rate of 1.8 children per couple.

8. 时间 表示时间的词有：when、before、after、since、now、later 等。

例 44 When we study the systematic evolution of lung and skin and hair of living things from protein to unicellular creatures to developed multicellular animals, vertebrate animals（脊椎动物）and human beings, we have found the internal relation of "the lung is connected with skin and hair".

例 45 After three cases that reported scant information were excluded, we examined the clinical features and safety of the hypersensitivity reaction induced by the challenge test using Kampo medicine in six cases.

例 46 In 1971, Folkman reported the theory of angiopoiesis（血管形成）, which states that if there is no blood vessel, tumor diameters（直径）will not exceed 3. Since then, a great deal of research has been focused on anti-angiogenic therapies.

9. 顺序 表示顺序的连接词有：first、second、finally、then、next 等。

例 47 There are limitations and future research questions to be tested in the Yin-DQ1. First, the Yin-DQ1 may not be sufficient to replace the individualized differential TCM diagnosis by an experienced practitioner.

例 48 Diminishment in moistening is exhibited by emaciation（消瘦）, dry mouth and/or throat and decreased amount of urine with yellowish color, while diminishment in calming leads to relative hyperactivity of yang, thus exhibiting deficiency-agitation and insomnia. Finally, diminishment of yang-heat controlling functions prevents yin from controlling yang, thus leading to hyperactivity of yang, i. e. irritable fever on palms and soles, tidal fever, reddened tongue, and weak and frequent pulse.

（姚秋慧）

第二节 常见句法错误

一、拼接句

两个或两个以上的独立句连接在一起，但是中间没有使用标点符号或错误地使用了逗号，这样形成的句子叫拼接句。拼接句的出现主要是由于标点符号的错误使用引起的。

例 1 误：Clinical data of 74 cases of unilateral total knee replacement（单侧全膝关节置换术）were retrospectively analyzed they were divided into two groups according to whether there was early continuous passive movement（CPM）（持续被动运动）exercises after operation.

分析：上句由 Clinical data of 74 cases of unilateral total knee replacement were retrospectively analyzed 和 they were divided into two groups according to whether there was early continuous passive movement（CPM）exercises after operation 两个独立句组成。这两个句子之间是并列关

系,因此它们之间应该使用表示并列关系的标点符号。

通常情况下,拼接句有以下三种改法:句子之间加上句号(后面句子的首字母需要大写),分号,或逗号加上并列连词 and、but、or、yet 等。

正:Clinical data of 74 cases of unilateral total knee replacement were retrospectively analyzed. They were divided into two groups according to whether there was early continuous passive movement(CPM)exercise after operation.

或:...were retrospectively analyzed;they were divided into...

或:...were retrospectively analyzed,and they were divided into...

二、句子片段

句子片段是指所表述的句子结构不完整,缺少必要的成分,如主语、谓语、宾语或补语等。这样的句子不符合语法规范,导致表意不清。

例 2　误:523 nurses from 5 hospitals with questionnaire to investigate the causes of adverse events.

分析:句子的主语是 523 nurses from 5 hospitals,后面缺少谓语动词,导致句子结构不完整,表意不清。

正:523 nurses from 5 hospitals were surveyed with questionnaire to investigate the causes of adverse events.

例 3　误:Furthermore,there are 1,724 authors be mentioned,among whom,1,331 published 1 paper,accounting for 77.2% of the total number of authors.

分析:分析句子结构可知,主句是一个包含 there be 句型的句子,因此 be mentioned 应该在句中充当定语,修饰前面的名词 authors。故 authors 后面应该加上 who 来引导定语从句,或者把 mentioned 前面的 be 去掉,mentioned 做后置定语。

正:Furthermore,there are 1,724 authors who were mentioned,among whom,1,331 published 1 paper,accounting for 77.2% of the total number of authors.

或:Furthermore,there are 1,724 authors mentioned,among whom...

三、赘述

学术论文的语言特征之一是行文简洁,目的是使读者能够快速、高效地获取信息。因此,应该尽量使用简洁的措辞,避免赘述。

例 4　误:Due to the fact that the direct measurements of the radical current(自由基电流)distribution cannot be performed at present,it is therefore complicated to describe in a detailed way the current build-up period for large machines like ours.

分析:分析句子结构可知,due to 引导原因状语,其中又含有 that 引导的同位语从句,结构比较复杂;主句是比较复杂的 it is+participle+to do 结构。因此,整个句子在阅读和理解上都比较费时费力。

正:Therefore, the detailed description of the current build-up period for large machines like ours is complicated due to the lack of direct measurements of the radical current distribution.

例 5 误:Our purpose is to investigate the nursing accidents of nurses in 5 hospitals and to analyze the causes of nursing accidents to provide references for the improvement of nursing safety control.

分析:句子中,to investigate 和 to analyze 两个表语可以合二为一,to provide references 和 control 可以省略。

正:Our purpose is to investigate and analyze the causes of nursing accidents in 5 hospitals for the improvement of nursing safety.

四、句式杂糅

句式杂糅是指把不同的句法结构放在等同的位置上,结果造成语句结构混乱、语义纠缠。

例 6 误:Intravenous(进入静脉的)administration of MB partly reversed the pulmonary vasodilator effect(肺血管扩张效应)of inhaled NO;MPAP increased from 2.0 kPa ± 0.6 kPa to 2.3 kPa ± 0.7 kPa. Cardiac(心脏的)output increased significantly.

分析:这句话中,作者要表达的意思是静脉内应用 MB 后,吸入一氧化氮的肺血管扩张效应得到了部分的逆转,表现在 MPAP(一种动脉压)升高和心输出量增加。第一个句子的两个分句在形式上并列,但含义上不并列。第二个分句和第二个句子都是肺血管扩张效应得到部分逆转的表现,因此应该是并列的。因此,第一个句子的第一个分句应独立成句,第二个分句和第二个句子构成并列句,对前者做进一步解释说明。

正:After intravenous administration of MB, the pulmonary vasodilating effect of NO inhaled was partly reversed. MPAP elevated from 2.0 kPa ± 0.6 kPa to 2.3 kPa ± 0.7 kPa, and cardiac output significantly increased.

例 7 误:In this paper, an improved MTT method was used to evaluate the antitumor activity of 15 new complexes of both two functional groups(dinuclear)and compared with that of the mononuclear complexes.

分析:就作者的本意而言,compared 的主语应是 the antitumor activity,但例句中 an improved MTT method 是全句的主语,有两个并列谓语,即 was used to evaluate the antitumor activity 和(was)compared with that of the mononuclear complexes。该长句结构不合理,造成歧义。应将 the antitumor activity 置于句首作主语,并相应调整句子其他部分。

正:In this paper, the antitumor activity of 15 new complexes of both two functional groups(dinuclear)was evaluated with an improved MTT method and compared with that of the mononuclear complexes.

五、逻辑关系混乱

在一些结构比较复杂的句子中,各个成分(如主语、谓语、表语等)之间的逻辑关系容易出现错误。

例 8 误:So it should be careful to administer methylene blue(亚甲蓝)for patients with pulmonary hypertension(肺动脉高压)during NO inhalation therapy.

分析:本句中 it 是形式主语,真正的主语是后面的动词不定式,即 to administer...should be careful,主语和表语的逻辑关系出现错误,careful 的逻辑主语应该是人,而不是动词不定式。

正:So methylene blue should be administered carefully for patients with pulmonary hypertension during NO inhalation therapy.

例 9 误:Fever longer than 10 days with large amount of pleural effusion and large patch of shadow on chest is significantly higher than control.

分析:从形式上看,这是一个比较句,其主干是 fever is significantly higher than control。但主语 fever 和 control 不是同一类事物,无法进行比较。

正:The occurrence of fever longer than 10 days with large amount of pleural effusion and large patch of shadow on chest is significantly higher than that in control group.

六、连词的误用

连词连接词语或句子,分为并列连词(用于连接两个并列成分)和从属连词(用于引导从句)两类。

例 10 误:The tiger population decreased dramatically because of their habitat was destroyed.

分析:because of 后面可以接原因状语,但不能引导从句。因此 because of 应该改为 because。

正:The tiger population decreased dramatically because their habitat was destroyed.

例 11 误:Ceramics(陶瓷)not only conducts electricity but also gases conduct electricity at low voltages.

分析:句子想要表达的意思是,"陶瓷和气体都会在低压下导电",整个句子由 not only...but also... 来连接。Not only...but also... 是并列连词,连接两个并列成分,如并列的主语、谓语等。

正:Not only ceramics but also gases conduct electricity at low voltages.

练习

1. 请分析下列句子属于哪种类型:simple sentence,compound sentence,complex sentence,compound-complex sentence。

(1) The purpose of this paper is to analyze the possible causes of the spatial differences.

（2）We have to admit that Heaven and Earth can be represented by the eight entities, four cosmic elements and four cosmic qualities.

（3）Nevertheless, this is the problem before us and we have to discuss a few popular charms.

（4）Traditional Chinese medicine（TCM）works on the premise that the human body has various forms of energy, or "Qi"（pronounced "chee"）, which flow through a series of well-defined tracts on the limbs, trunk and face.

（5）The result is that however desirable it may be to treat asthmatics with acupuncture at 3:00 in the morning, the treatment will invariably be performed during working hours.

（6）Lycium, as well as Jatropha extracts, seemed to be able to initiate cellular pathways that led to apoptosis when added to tumoral cells, but they did not show a significant cytotoxicity in contact with normal cells.

2. 请选择恰当的词或词组完成句子。

（1）＿＿＿＿（Furthermore/In addition to）the refinement of cryopreservation protocols, more attention should also be paid to the physiological factors affecting cryopreservation success, such as the recovery phase.

（2）＿＿＿＿（Therefore/Although）, they can be quickly categorized as cavity-type zeolites. ＿＿＿＿（While/In contrast）, the other three zeolites presented in Figure 9 are of channel-type structures, in which the widths of the connecting pathways are about the same size as the largest cavities.

（3）Metals have many free-moving electrons. ＿＿＿＿（Consequently/Since）metals are good conductors of heat.

（4）CVI was significantly higher at forest edges ＿＿＿＿（however/while）CSI peaked at the furthest point from forest edge.

（5）Prior to human logging activities, 85%—95% of the land surface had been covered by forest ecosystems. ＿＿＿＿（Hence/Since）, forest structures and tree characteristics are of crucial significance for the conservation of large-scale biodiversity.

（6）Hochuekkito increases titers of influenza virus-specific IgA antibody and total IgA antibody in the nasal cavity. ＿＿＿＿（Furthermore/As a result）, Hochuekkito inhibits rhinovirus infection in human tracheal epithelial cells, by decreasing intercellular adhesion molecule-1 levels, and blocks viral RNA from entering the cytoplasm via the airway epithelial cell endosomes.

（7）These measures have not been implemented ＿＿＿＿（due to/because）potentially even greater compression can be achieved to address the current problem by resorting to a high-resolution stable scanner.

(8) Factors _____ (such as/likewise) agricultural extension, formal education, and the nutritional status of households were found to have a statistically significant relationship with reducing technical inefficiency.

3. 请根据句意重新排列下列句子的顺序。

(1) However, aspirin is also associated with bleeding. Patients are often asked to stop taking aspirin before bronchoscopy to reduce the risk of bleeding.

(2) We compared the number and severity of bleeding events in those taking aspirin with those who were not and determined that aspirin does not increase the risk of bleeding.

(3) The effectiveness of this practice has never been tested.

(4) In patients with atherosclerotic vascular disease, aspirin is recommended to prevent myocardial infarction and graft occlusion.

(5) Thus, we sought to determine whether aspirin really does increase the risk of bleeding after bronchoscopy.

4. 请找出下列句子中的错误并修改。

(1) Australian education centers will require a broad communication network, inefficiencies will otherwise occur.

(2) Service costs to prospective students should be kept to a minimum educational fees are already expensive.

(3) Using RT-PCR to clone and sequence IL-12 p40cDNA from the RNA extracted from cord blood dentritic cells (DC) of newborns in Beijing, China.

(4) Notably, both ES cells and iPS cells had not been infected with a carcinogenic virus.

(5) The specificity analysis demonstrated that hybridization did not occur between nucleotide sequences with a single-base mismatch, which is partly consistent with what Thomas Naiser and E. Lorenzo has reported. (Loreno *et al.*, 2008; Naiser *et al.*, 2008)

(6) The election campaign is in its final stages two candidates remain.

(7) Measurements of blood pH were made with a capillary electrode.

(8) Changes of the refraction angle as a result of nucleic acid hybirdization were recorded in real time and then converted to electrical signals and further to the concentration of analytes by the system software.

5. 请把下列句子中的汉语翻译成英语。

(1) _____ (如表所示) in figure 1, about 83% of the younger groups are in favor of personal development and promotion.

(2) Personality traits _____ (可能与······有关)to the various aspects of environmental concern.

(3) _____ (我们比较了)the chemical composition of wile-type PG with PG isolated from PBP1a or LpoALpoB cells.

(4) There were no _____ (显著差异)favoring either strategy in any predefined subgroup.

(5) _____ (众所周知)cancers arise from a series of sequential mutations that occur as a result of genetic instability and environmental factors.

(6) We also find statistical evidence that _____ (这些类似性是因为)RNA editing.

（姚秋慧）

第四章 标 点

一篇结构清楚、表意准确的英语论文必须正确使用标点符号。误用或滥用标点符号会影响读者对论文结构和内容的理解。本章着重介绍英语论文写作中常用的标点符号,包括句号、逗号、冒号、引号、括号、分号、破折号、连字符、所有格符号、问号等。

第一节 标点的使用

一、句号(Period)

句号在英语和汉语中的表达功能相同,均表明一句话到此结束。在形式上两者有所区别,英语表示为".",而汉语则表示为"。"。

（一）分割完整的句子

在英语写作中,句号主要用来表明句子意思的完结。

例1 TCM was developed through thousands of years of empirical testing and refinement.

例2 Equally clear is the fact that these compounds have no direct effect on the human body because the gut cannot absorb them.

（二）缩写

除用来结束句子外,英语缩写中也会使用句号。如果缩写由小写字母构成或者由大小写字母混合构成,需要使用句号,例如:a. m.,etc.,vol.,Inc.,Jr.,Mrs. 。如果缩写由大写字母构成,则需要省略句号,例如:AIDS,BBC,NBC,CNNIAEA,NATO,NBC。

句号在缩写的使用中存在特殊情况。一些科技用语的缩写会省略句号,例如:kHz(kilohertz),rpm(revolutions per minute),kg(kilogram),Na(sodium)。而一些大写字母构成的缩写,特别是学位用语,却使用句号,例如:J. D. (Juris Doctor),D. D. S. (Doctor of Dental Surgery)。

如果在句末出现缩写且带有句号,句子不需要再添加句号。

例3 He is a manager at Ess Technology Inc.

例4 Mary said that they would continue the project at 9:00 a. m.

二、逗号(Comma)

在英语写作中,逗号的用法相对繁杂,往往让人感觉困惑。误用或滥用逗号容易导致误解语义,因此在写作中要注意正确使用。

（一）列举

逗号可以用来分隔列举的若干条目。通常用 and 连接最后两个条目,并且 and 之前可以添加逗号。

例 5　The TCM doctor then listens to the patient's voice to see if there are any breathing problems, cough or phlegm, and sniffs to detect any body odors that might indicate ill health.

例 6　The highly valued plant is mainly used to treat jaundice, heart pain, and dysentery.

例 7　We therefore suggest that dissecting the mode of action of clinically effective formulae at the molecular, cellular, and organism levels may be a good strategy in exploring the value of traditional medicine.

（二）并列句

并列句由两个或两个以上的独立分句构成,分句之间由并列连词连接。常用的并列连词有 and、but 和 or。并列句的分句之间用逗号连接,且并列连词之前添加逗号。

例 8　Kampo medicine shares many similarities with TCM: they both support the concept of a gradual improvement in the body's condition using natural agents, and diagnosis is made using a pattern of symptoms.

例 9　In these countries, different traditional medicines might use different prescriptions or methods of diagnosis, but the underlying philosophy and principles are similar because they all originate in China.

（三）同位语

逗号常用于分隔中心词与同位语。

例 10　The use of rhino horn dates back to at least 1,800 years ago and is referenced in *Shennong's Classic of Materia Medica*, the very first book of Chinese herbal medicine, says Huijun Shen, president of the UK Association of Traditional Chinese Medicine in London.

例 11　Adam Smith, science and communications officer for the Alliance for Natural Health International (ANHI) in Dorking, United Kingdom, a non-governmental campaign group promoting the use of herbal medicines and other approaches to healthcare, fears that patients will lose out on some Asian medicines because they have not been used in Europe for the requisite 15 years, even though they have been consumed in East Asia for a considerably longer period.

例 12　The major classic of TCM, the *Internal Classic of the Yellow Emperor*, says that the stone needle was developed by the ethnic group living on the eastern side of China.

（四）非限制性定语从句

非限制性定语从句仅是对先行词的附加说明,对先行词本身不起限定作用。如果去掉这一从句,剩下部分的语义依然完整。先行词和非限制性定语从句之间需要用逗号隔开。

例 13　Despite growing support among the Japanese public, Kampo is eclipsed by Western medicine, which accounts for 98% of total pharmaceutical production in Japan.

例 14　Together, these data suggest that CCPA acts locally, probably on unmyelinated C fibers in the superficial peroneal nerve, which travels in close proximity to the Zusanli points.

（五）导入成分

逗号可以用来分隔句首的导入成分和句子的主干部分。导入成分可以是从句、短语或单词。

1. 从句　从句通常用来引出主句,往往使用下列词语来引导:after, although, as, because, before, if, since, though, until, when。如果从句出现在主句之后,一般无需添加逗号。

例 15　Because the two have many things in common, it may be worthwhile to carry out a comparative study of the traditional medical education in Japan and South Korea.

例 16　Various measures were taken to protect and conserve Korean herbal medicine when foreign medicinal herbs were being imported.

2. 短语　常见的导入短语有介词短语、分词短语、不定式短语和独立主格结构。

例 17　After taking it for several days, the patient was able to stand and walk again.

例 18　Taking functional dyspepsia as an example, the study aimed to establish and analyze the evolution model of TCM pathogenesis.

例 19　To study the cause of the disease, 500 cases were investigated.

例 20　The sun radiating intense heat, we sought shelter in the shopping mall.

注意:如果介词短语少于四个单词,可以使用也可不使用逗号。

例 21　At that time, TCM spread to Japan and began to develop independently.

At that time TCM spread to Japan and began to develop independently.

3. 词语　通常在导入词和句子主干之间添加逗号来加以分隔。导入词一般是副词,例如:however, meanwhile, furthermore, still。

例 22　Consequently, some traditional herbal products had been available to patients without the quality and safety guarantees that come with registration.

例 23　However, academic scientists and the pharmaceutical industry have not been very successful at isolating the active substances in TCM preparations.

三、冒号（Colon）

冒号主要用于列举、解释说明和强调。

1. 列举　冒号通常用来引出列举的内容,且冒号之前需是语义和结构完整的句子。

例 24　In addition, the WHO has established 25 collaborating centers for traditional medicine: 7 in China, 5 in Africa, 3 in Europe, 2 in each of Japan, South Korea, India and the United States, and 1 in both North Korea and Vietnam.

例 25　The following positively charged residues have been identified to be important for PIP_2 interaction: R67, K188Q, and R216.

2. 解释说明　一个句子中,如果第二个分句用来解释说明第一个分句,那么两个分句之间用冒号连接。也适用于这一用法标题的写作，即主标题和副标题之间用冒号连接。

例 26 Part of Kampo's problem is institutional：unlike China and South Korea，where governments promote traditional medicine，Japan has neither government departments nor public institutes dedicated to Kampo.

例 27 The experimental development of the new technology made possible a new tool：a detector with less energy consumption.

例 28 Convergence：Where West meets East

3. 强调　在句子结尾处，冒号可以用来强调特定的词或短语。

例 29 After three weeks of data analysis，the decisive factor for the experiment results was：age.

四、引号（Quotation Mark）

（一）基本使用规则

1. 若引用的内容置于句首，则引用内容的结尾处需在引号内添加逗号，整句话的结尾处加句号。

例 30 "The medical practice of TCM is a process of trial and error，and concerns the understanding and control of herbs from the Chinese materia medica，" says Daqing Zhang，director of the Center for History of Medicine at Peking University in Beijing.

例 31 "We've done some work showing that herbal medicines produce notable shifts in gut microbial metabolism，and those shifts can be quite stable over quite long periods of time，" Nicholson says.

如果其后紧跟另外一句完整的引用，则该引用部分首字母大写，句号放在引号内。

例 32 "Some of these medicines have been around for thousands of years，" explains Dick Middleton，technical director at Schwabe Pharma UK in Buckinghamshire. "If they didn't work they would have disappeared by now."

例 33 "Because these complex diseases have multifocal problems，no single drug can treat them，" says Jeremy Nicholson，a biochemist at Imperial College London. "Chinese medicine is a polypharmacy，with multiple synergistically active compounds in the mixtures；the reason some of the medicines probably work is that they drug multiple targets at the same time."

2. 一般情况下，逗号或句号放置在引号内。

例 34 The author suggested，"The basic structure of biological membrane is determined by the substance，and proteins provide nutrition for most functions of the membrane."

如果引用的完整的一句话被中途打断，则前半句的逗号放在第一对引号内，下半句的首字母不用大写，句号放在第二对引号内。

例 35 "If we can start to unravel how TCM works，" he says，"it might offer a completely new horizon on how you drug the human body."

例 36 "I never used them，even when they were legal，" he recalls，"because they were so expensive."

3. 引号可用于标注短篇故事、短篇诗歌、散文、章节、歌曲、电视节目等。

例 37 "The Fall of the House of Usher" by Edgar Allan Poe

例 38 "An Essay on Dream" by Thomas Paine

例 39 "Hey Jude" by The Beatles

（二）引出标点的选择

通常引用内容前使用的标点符号主要有三种情况：逗号、冒号和无标点。

1. **逗号** 如果引用的内容单独成句，则在引号前加逗号。

例 40 So, much like ginseng, "it is most likely they work by changing gut microbiota."

2. **冒号** 引用内容之前的导入句本身是一个完整的句子，则在引号前加冒号。

例 41 The current World Health Organization definition of the term is based on a 1948 consensus: "A state of complete physical, mental, and social well-being and not merely the absence of disease or infirmity."

3. **不使用标点** 如果引用的内容已糅合于整个句子，则引号前不添加任何标点。

例 42 However, working the other way around—starting with a complex herbal mixture and trying to "deconvolute the synergy"—is tough, says Lee.

例 43 The THMPD "aims to protect public health and at the same time secure the free movement of herbal products within the EU", according to the European Medicines Agency.

五、括号（Parenthesis）

写作中通常使用括号来增补文章信息。括号内的信息可以是单词、短语或完整的句子，并且括号内的内容不影响原句的结构完整和语义表达。括号的正确使用与逗号或句号的位置密切相关。

1. **内容不单独成句** 如果括号出现在句末，且括号内的内容不单独成句，则句号放在括号外。

例 44 TCM encompasses a wide range of practices, including some that are familiar to the West, such as herbal medicine and acupuncture, plus others that remain peculiar to most Westerners, such as cupping (heated cup therapy), tuina (massage), qigong (movement and breathing exercises), and moxibustion (burnt mugwort therapy).

例 45 Although the concept might seem strange to Western perceptions, many TCM practitioners draw a parallel with the well-understood scientific concepts of metabolism (roughly equivalent to energy), immunity, and homeostasis (balance).

例 46 The mean number of days with pain was decreased by half (from 21 to 10 d/mo).

2. **内容单独成句** 如果括号内是完整的句子，则句号放在括号内，且括号外不需要再添加句号。

例 47 It is estimated that there are at least half of all the Chinese TCM patents aimed for package design, rather than for the drug itself. (There are not any official figures.)

例 48　The idea that theoretical physics can be taught without reference to complex mathematics is patently absurd. (But don't tell that to the publishers of such mathematics-free books—or the people who buy them.)

3. 位于句子中部　括号出现在长句的中部，则紧随其后的标点符号应该放在括号外。

例 49　Concepts include yin and yang, which represent opposing yet complementary essences of nature; wuxing, which covers the five basic elements of the universe (wood, fire, earth, metal, and water); qi or energy; and xue, the blood.

例 50　This perspective has, of course, long been central to the concept of health in traditional Chinese medicine (TCM), which further includes spiritual fulfillment and a sense of individual well-being.

例 51　In the process of purifying and testing the antimalarial agent artemisinin, phytochemist Youyou Tu realized that the age-old Chinese technique of boiling and high-temperature extraction destroys the artemisinin contained in *Artemisia annua* (qinghao in Chinese), a herb used in traditional Chinese medicine (TCM) for hundreds of years.

六、分号（Semicolon）

分号和句号或逗号的功能类似，主要用于分割长句或连接若干成分。通常认为分号的使用效力小于句号，但要大于逗号。

1. 并列句　如果省略并列句中的并列连词，则使用分号来连接分句。

例 52　Some countries did not regulate traditional herbs at all; others classified herbal products as food supplements rather than medicines, and so subjected them to less scrutiny.

2. 过渡表达方式连接的分句　如果两个分句之间以过渡词或短语连接，则在过渡词或短语前添加分号。过渡词或短语包括：accordingly、consequently、for example、nevertheless、so、thus 等。

例 53　These bugs have been linked with a number of health benefits in the human host; in particular, they can modulate the immune system in ways known to reduce the risk of autoimmune diseases such as diabetes mellitus type 1 (ref. 1).

3. 并列成分　两个或两个以上并列词组或分句之间可以用分号连接，分句或词组中往往有逗号。

例 54　The rhino and its horn are not alone: powdered tiger bone is used to treat rheumatism; the scales of the toothless, anteater-like pangolin are believed to reduce swelling and improve blood circulation; and Guilinggao, a jelly derived from the shells of freshwater turtles, was used to treat smallpox in a nineteenth-century emperor, with little success—in Taiwan it is now reputed to cure cancer.

例 55　Abbreviations: K2P, two-P domain K$^+$ channel; CFTR, cystic fibrosis transmembrane conductance regulator；RyR，ryanodine receptor；NCX，sodium/calcium exchanger.

例 56　Next，the practitioner questions how the patient feels overall：if they are hot or cold；whether they are sweating；how their stools look；if the patient is thirsty，and so forth.

七、破折号（Dash）

破折号在英语写作中可以起到解释、承接和概括的作用。

1. 解释说明　破折号可以用来承接上文和解释说明。

例 57　Traditional Herbal Medicine at Kashima Rosai Hospital in Kamisu reported 503 cases of side effects out of 2,530 total prescriptions，with symptoms varying from poor appetite to 26 cases of liver disorder—half of which were caused by herbal medicine（4 in 1,000 cases）.

例 58　China only started awarding patents for TCM products in the 1990s，and there are still no specific standards that govern whether a particular TCM formula is eligible for a patent—the same rules also govern food recipes，for example.

2. 总体概括　破折号也可用来总结概括上文列举的条目或内容。

例 59　Ion channels，transporters，cytoskeleton remodeling，and vesicle trafficking—many cellular functions are regulated by PIP_2.

八、连字符（Hyphen）

在英语写作中，连字符的主要功能是构造特定的复合词。

1. 复合名词　连字符的构词功能主要体现在：连接两个或两个以上的单词构成新的复合名词，例如：well-being，by-product，pain-killer。连字符还可以连接大写字母和名词来构成新单词，例如：X-ray，U-turn，G-protein，U-wave，ST-segment，M-cell。

2. 复合形容词　连字符可用来连接两个或两个以上的单词或词素构成新的复合形容词。连字符可以连接两个或多个单词，例如：short-term treatment，above-mentioned therapies，well-understood concepts，well-known plant，up-to-date style。连字符也可以连接单词和词缀，例如：anti-inflammatory，anti-diabetic，anti-hyperglycemic，non-linear，non-bacterial，self-inflicted，cancer-related，AIDS-related，smoke-free，noise-free，panic-stricken，cancer-stricken。

九、所有格符号（Apostrophe）

所有格符号主要有两项用途：缩写和表明所属关系。所有格符号表示缩写的现象非常普遍，例如：is not 缩写成 isn't。所有格符号用于表明所属关系时有以下几种情况：

1. 单数名词和不定代词后加"'s"，如 someone's experiment。

2. 以 s 结尾的复数名词加"'"，如 five years' experience。

3. 不以 s 结尾的复数名词加"'s"，如 the women's desks。

十、问号（Question Mark）

鉴于学术论文写作的专业性和严谨性，行文中并不常用到问号。但撰写论文的标题或小标题时，可以使用问号来强化主题。

例 60　And likewise，can new perspectives being advanced in the West，such as systems biology，help lay a scientific foundation for TCM?

例 61　Can Duhuo Jisheng decoction be applied for knee osteoarthritis?

例 62　Psychological counseling in cancer pain：is it a more liberal approach?

（邱冬）

第二节　标点使用的常见错误

一、形式差异错误

英汉两种语言的标点在形式上存在差异，这导致英语学习者在写作中误用汉语标点符号。英汉标点的形式差异主要表现在以下方面：

1. 英语中没有书名号，汉语的书名号为"《 》"　英语写作中提及各类作品的名称时，通常使用斜体来表示。

2. 英语中没有顿号，汉语中的顿号为"、"　英语写作中需要列举时，通常会使用逗号分隔列举的条目。

3. 英语中的省略号是行底的连续三个英语句号"..."　汉语中的省略号是居中的六个圆点，即"……"。

二、句号

1. 一"句"到底　一"句"到底容易导致句子逻辑混乱，阅读困难。因此，撰写论文时要善于利用句号分割长句，确保语义流畅通顺。

例 1　误：For temperatures below 10℃，the four bacteria examined had about the same reproductive delay when the reproductive delay was defined as the time to complete a reproductive cycle，in spite of the large variations in reproductive delay among the four bacteria at higher temperatures.

正：The reproductive delay was defined as the time to complete a reproductive cycle. The four bacteria examined had about the same reproductive delay for temperatures below 10℃，in spite of the large variations in reproductive delay among the four bacteria at higher temperatures.

2. 缩写问题　滥用或误用缩写会使读者难以正确理解句子意思。

例 2　误：Figure 1-1 shows a gamma-ray line，i. e.，radiation at a single gamma-ray energy level, that theorists had predicted would result from <u>N. Cygni</u>.

正：Figure 1-1 shows a gamma-ray line（radiation at a single gamma-ray energy level）that theorists had predicted would result from <u>Nova Cygni</u>.

三、逗号

1. 逗号粘连　指用逗号连接两个或两个以上语义独立、形式完整的句子，而两个句子之间没有相应的连词。此类错误会使读者很难理清句子之间的逻辑关系，极易导致曲解或误解句子含义。

例 3　误：Rats were sacrificed on day 7 after treatment with cisplatin<u>,</u>the serum level of cisplatin was determined by flow cytometry.

正：Rats were sacrificed on day 7 after treatment with cisplatin<u>.</u> The serum level of cisplatin was determined by flow cytometry.

2. 滥用逗号　滥用逗号会导致句子的语义不清，使读者断句困难。

例 4　误：As determined by ANOVA multi-group comparison test, unsupervised hierarchical clustering was performed<u>,</u>on a subset of 85 significant genes, and the genes themselves<u>,</u>were expressed differently<u>,</u>among cell line groups.

正：As determined by ANOVA multi-group comparison test, unsupervised hierarchical clustering was <u>performed on</u> a subset of 85 significant genes, and the genes <u>themselves were</u> expressed <u>differently among</u> cell line groups.

3. 导入成分问题　逗号通常添加在导入词和句子主干之间，起到分隔的作用。

例 5　误：<u>Interestingly the</u> therapy has been welcomed for more than 2,500 years in TCM through several means.

正：<u>Interestingly, the</u> therapy has been welcomed for more than 2,500 years in TCM through several means.

若从句出现在主句之后，一般无需添加逗号。

例 6　误：Therefore, practitioners should be cautious<u>, when</u> applying White Tiger Decoction Plus Ginseng in medical practice.

正：Therefore, practitioners should be <u>cautious when</u> applying White Tiger Decoction Plus Ginseng in medical practice.

4. 定语从句问题　非限制性定语从句的先行词和从句之间要以逗号隔开，而限制性定语从句则不需要。

例 7　误：The medical <u>tradition which</u> was mainly advocated from the 13th to 15th <u>century referred</u> to the active integration of local herbal medicine with medical knowledge from China.

正：The medical tradition<u>, </u>which was mainly advocated from the 13th to 15th century<u>, </u>referred to the active integration of local herbal medicine with medical knowledge from China.

例 7 中 which 引导的非限制性定语从句是插入成分，所以需要以逗号隔开从句和主句的剩余部分。

四、冒号

冒号可以用来列举条目，但是冒号之前必须是语义和结构完整的句子。

例 8 误：Several characteristics of Hyangyak Medicine are：locally cultivated herbs，limited numbers of drugs，and raw or fresh materials.

正：Studies have found out several characteristics of Hyangyak Medicine：locally cultivated herbs，limited numbers of drugs，and raw or fresh materials.

例 8 冒号之前不是完整的句子，不符合冒号的使用规则，因此对冒号前的部分进行修改，使其独立成句。

五、破折号

滥用破折号会使文章不够流畅连贯，影响读者对文章逻辑和意思的把握。行文中可以通过调整语序、改写为从句、改换其他标点符号等方式进行修改。

例 9 误：Traditional medicine—a system of ancient medical practice that differs in substance，methodology，and philosophy from modern medicine—plays an important role in health maintenance for the peoples of Asia，and is becoming more frequently used in countries in the West.

正：As a system of ancient medical practice that differs in substance，methodology，and philosophy from modern medicine，traditional medicine plays an important role in health maintenance for the peoples of Asia，and is becoming more frequently used in countries in the West.

例 10 误：But Kampo—imported from China 1,500 years ago—is under pressure.

正：But Kampo that was imported from China 1,500 years ago is under pressure.

六、引号

1. 引号内的标点使用 直接引用的内容放在句首，则引用的部分要在引号内加逗号。

例 11 误："You can use different drugs or approaches，but all drugs and treatment strategies have to pass the same standards to show that they are effective" says Rao.

正："You can use different drugs or approaches，but all drugs and treatment strategies have to pass the same standards to show that they are effective，" says Rao.

2. 引出标点的使用 如果导入句本身单独成句，则需要在引号前使用冒号。如果引用的内容是完整的句子，则需要在引号前使用逗号。

例 12 误：Toshihiko Hanawa，director-general of Kitasato University Oriental Medicine Research Center，adds："And for Japan，it is imperative that we establish a government support system."

正：Toshihiko Hanawa，director-general of Kitasato University Oriental Medicine Research Center，adds，"And for Japan，it is imperative that we establish a government support system."

例 12 中的导入部分不能独立成句,故不能使用冒号导出。引用部分可以单独成句,所以改为使用逗号引出。

练习

请为下列句子添加标点。

(1) Conversely abnormal social interactions are debilitating symptoms of several neuropsychiatric disorders notably autism spectrum disorder ASD

(2) To examine whether 5HT release in the NAc shares these features we performed two assays real time conditioned placed preference CPP and optogenetic intracranial self-stimulation

(3) These behavioural effects of 5HT in the NAc are markedly different from the acute reinforcing properties of the release of dopamine in the NAc suggesting critical differences in the NAc circuitry modulation by which these major neuromodulators mediate their behavioural effects

(4) Adding or removing an ingredient sometimes doesn't much change the efficacy of a compound TCM prescription says Kaixian Chen president of the Shanghai University of Traditional Chinese Medicine

(5) For example strain M which had been subjected to *in vivo* passaging and drug treatment was the most genetically distinct the 11 strains used by the connectivity map project 16 over a 10-year period clustered tightly together and sibling strains D and E which were only a few passages apart were the closest to each other

(6) The MCF7 HT29 MDAM 453 and A375 cell lines were cultured in RPMI 1640

(7) All strains of the same cell line were cultured under the same conditions cell identity was confirmed and the cells were confirmed to be mycoplasma free

(8) There is obviously an essential difference between a TCM formula and other compound products says Song The concept of fangyi is unique to TCM prescriptions and should be protected by the patent law

(9) There are millions of crocodiles in the world Zain observes but only a few thousand tigers

(10) The expression of 222 miRNA precursors was profiled in 32 commonly used cell lines of lung breast head and neck colorectal prostate pancreatic and hematopoietic cancers

(邱冬)

参 考 文 献

----

[1] ATTELE A S,ZHOU Y P,XIE J T,et al. Antidiabetic effects of Panax ginseng berry extract and the identification of an effective component[J]. Diabetes,2002,51(6):1851-1858.

[2] NGWAI Y B,IZEBE K S,IJELE I G,et al. Seropositivity of *Chlamydophila pneumoniae* immunoglobulin G antibody of HIV/AIDS patients in Abuja,Nigeria[J]. Asian Pacific Journal of Tropical Medicine,2010(8): 666-668.

[3] BROWN T M,HALLIDAY M A K,MCINTOSH A,et al. The linguistic sciences and language teaching[J]. The Modern Language Review,1967,62(1):106-107.

[4] CAO J,ZHANG J,WANG Z,et al. Hypothyroidism as a potential biomarker of efficacy of famitinib,a novel VEGFR-2 inhibitor in metastatic breast cancer[J]. Cancer Chemotherapy and Pharmacology,2014,74(2): 389-398.

[5] GILBERT N. Regulations:Herbal medicine rule book[J]. Nature,2011,480(7378):S98-S99.

[6] VAN DER GREEF J. Perspective:All systems go[J]. Nature,2011,480(7378):S87.

[7] FLOWERDEW J,PEACOCK M. Research perspectives on English for academic purposes[M]. Cambridge: Cambridge University Press,2011.

[8] KANG B H,PLESCIA J,DOHI T,et al. Regulation of tumor cell mitochondrial homeostasis by an organelle-specific Hsp90 chaperone network[J]. Cell,2007,131(2):257-270.

[9] LEE S,PARK J,LEE H,et al. Development and validation of yin-deficiency questionnaire[J]. American Journal of Chinese Medicine,2007,35(1):11-20.

[10] PALMA V,LIM D A,DAHMANE N,et al. Sonic hedgehog controls stem cell behavior in the postnatal and adult brain[J]. Development,2005,132(2):335-344.

[11] DAY R A,SAKADUSKI N. Scientific english:A guide for scientists and other professionals[M]. 3rd ed. Santa Barbara:Greenwood Press,2011.

[12] SAKURAI M. Perspective:herbal dangers[J]. Nature,2011,480(7378):S97.

[13] TAKAYAMA S,KANEKO S,NUMATA T,et al. Literature review:herbal medicine treatment after large-scale disasters[J]. American Journal of Chinese Medicine,2017,45(7):1345-1364:1-20.

[14] WALSH J J,CHRISTOFFEL D J,HEIFETS B D,et al. 5-HT release in nucleus accumbens rescues social deficits in mouse autism model[J]. Nature,2018,560(7720):589-594.

[15] WANG J F,CAI C Z,KONG C Y,et al. A Computer method for validating traditional Chinese medicine herbal prescriptions[J]. American Journal of Chinese Medicine,2005,33(2):281-297.

[16] WIDDOWSON H G. Learning purpose and language use[M]. Oxford:Oxford University Press,1983.

[17] ZHA L H,HE L S,LIAN F M,et al. Clinical strategy for optimal traditional Chinese medicine(TCM)herbal

dose selection in disease therapeutics：expert consensus on classic TCM herbal formula dose conversion［J］. The American Journal of Chinese Medicine，2015，43（8）：1515-1524.

［18］ZHANG J，ZHANG M，TANG W X，et al. Buckling of spherical shells subjected to external pressure：A comparison of experimental and theoretical data［J］. Thin Walled Structures，2017，111：58-64.

［19］蔡基刚.“学术英语”课程需求分析和教学方法研究［J］.外语教学理论与实践，2012（2）：30.

［20］蔡基刚.台湾成功大学从 EGP 向 ESP 转型的启示［J］.外语教学理论与实践，2013（3）：7-11.

［21］蔡基刚，廖雷朝.学术英语还是专业英语——我国大学 ESP 教学重新定位思考［J］.外语教学，2010，31（6）：47-50，73.

［22］陈彬彬. Internet 医学信息资源检索与利用的探讨［J］.电脑知识与技术，2016，12（21）：188-189.

［23］陈国琪.医学期刊刊名和人名的缩写及音译方法［J］.医学信息学杂志，2000，21（6）：53-55.

［24］陈纪国.医学论文的温哥华格式［J］.中山大学学报论丛，2002，22（3）：293-296.

［25］陈振华，邹雨轩.医学英语病句诊治［J］.泸州医学院学报，2013，36（6）：642-643.

［26］范华泉，冷怀明.浅析医学期刊来稿论文英文摘要中常见标点符号错误［J］.管理学家，2010（12）：377-378.

［27］范晓晖.论医学论文英文摘要中被动语态的滥用［J］.中国科技翻译，2005，18（4）：11-13.

［28］何康民.英语学术论文写作［M］.武汉：武汉大学出版社，2007.

［29］胡庚申.论文写作与国际发表［M］.北京：外语教学与研究出版社，2014.

［30］胡友珍，何小平，王志芳.英语学术论文写作教程［M］.北京：中国农业大学出版社，2011.

［31］黄燕.医学文献检索［M］.北京：人民卫生出版社，2009.

［32］黄正谷，李同心.医学文献的检索方法［J］.检验医学与临床，2014，11（9）：1293-1294.

［33］金坤林.如何撰写和发表 SCI 期刊论文［M］.北京：科学出版社，2008.

［34］鞠玉梅.国外 EAP 教学与研究概览［J］.外语教学，2006，27（2）：1-6.

［35］李丽君.英语学术论文及留学文书写作［M］.北京：清华大学出版社，北京交通大学出版社，2009.

［36］李向武.英语学术论文写作教程［M］.成都：西南交通大学出版社，2015.

［37］李振吉.中医药 SCI 论文写作与发表实用教材［M］.北京：人民卫生出版社，2013.

［38］廖荣霞.英文 SCI 生物医学论文写作教程［M］.北京：科学出版社，2012.

［39］刘新娟，刘翟，刘文勇.去美国读研究生［M］.北京：中国人民大学出版社，2014.

［40］刘彦哲.医学英语论文摘要阅读与写作［M］.上海：复旦大学出版社，2012.

［41］刘振聪，修月祯.英语学术论文写作［M］.北京：中国人民大学出版社，2013.

［42］刘志强.个人陈述文体写作中应注意的几个问题［J］.牡丹江大学学报，2007，16（4）：49-50.

［43］马莉.英语学术论文写作及语体风格［M］.北京：北京大学出版社，2011.

［44］王征爱，许瑾，宋建武.英语医学科技论文写作中的常见错误（Ⅱ）［J］.第一军医大学学报，2003，23（3）：284-288.

［45］文师吾，谢日华. SCI 医学英文论文的撰写与发表［M］.北京：人民卫生出版社，2012.

［46］吴江梅，黄佩娟.英语科技论文写作［M］.北京：中国人民大学出版社，2013.

［47］解景田，谢来华. SCI 攻略：生物医药科技论文的撰写与发表［M］.2 版.北京：科学出版社，2015.

［48］张学军.医学科研论文撰写与发表［M］.2 版.北京：人民卫生出版社，2014.

练习参考答案

中 篇

第二章 英文医学论文的结构与写作

第一节 文题

1. 请将下列文题改为主副文题的格式。

（1）A light and electron microscopic study of primary sarcoma of the heart：2 cases

（2）Laser surgery of the liver：an experimental study

（3）Clinical analysis of subacute thyroiditis：55 cases

（4）Evidence-based medicine：a new approach to teaching the practice of medicine

（5）Autophagy in cell death：an innocent convict？

2. 请将下列文题翻译成英语。

（1）TCM pathogenesis of tumor from the perspective of triple energizer qi transformation

（2）TCM syndrome distribution with acute exacerbation of chronic obstructive pulmonary disease：a report of 302 cases

（3）Metrology and visualization analysis of acupuncture and moxibustion related literature of Web of Science in the past 5 years by CiteSpace application

（4）System evaluation of traditional exercise therapy intervention on pain and joint function improvement in patients with knee osteoarthritis

（5）Clinical curative effect and safety of Danhong injection（丹红注射液）combined with routine therapy in treating patients suffering from cerebral infarction：a meta-analysis

第三节 摘要

练习1

请将下列句子翻译成英语。

（1）To analyze the content of active components in fresh Danshen（Radix Salviae Miltiorrhizae, Red Sage Root）from different producing areas, and assess reasonably the medicinal quality of fresh Danshen.

（2）To study the clinical efficacy of Qingshen granule, formulated by TCM therapy principle of clearing heat（qingre）, eliminating dampness（huashi）and removing blood stasis（quyu）, on chronic renal failure patients with damp-heat pattern.

（3）This N of 1, randomized controlled, double blind trial was designed to evaluate the clinical efficacy of Liuwei Dihuang capsule in the treatment of liver-kidney yin deficiency syndrome and to assess the applicability and reliability of this method in the evaluation of syndrome response.

练习 2

请将下列句子翻译成英语。

（1）A total of 282 patients eligible were divided into treatment group（n=136）and control group（n=146）. All patients were treated with conventional therapy; in addition, patients of treatment group took orally Qingshen granule for consecutive 12 weeks.

（2）Finally, we analyzed the patient population suitable for this therapy according to the relationship between the patients' body weight and curative effect.

（3）The content of 5 salvianolic acids and 12 tanshinones in fresh Danshen, from 7 different producing areas, were determined by applying LTQ-Orbitrap XL high-resolution mass spectrometer.

练习 3

请将下列句子翻译成英语。

（1）The content of active components in fresh Danshen from the same producing area were basically the same, and there was significant difference in content of active components among fresh Danshen from different producing areas.

（2）The total clinical effective rate of the treatment group（79.41%）was significantly higher than that of the control group（67.12%）, and there was significant difference between the two groups（P<0.05）.

（3）There was no statistical difference in the curative effect on urinary red cells and various indexes after a 12-week treatment between the two groups.

练习 4

请将下列句子翻译成英语。

（1）The result shows the efficacy and safety of traditional Chinese medicine on the treatment of patients with early diabetic nephropathy.

（2）N of 1 randomized controlled trials can be used to evaluate the therapeutic effect of syndrome-like Chinese medicines, and they are applicable and reliable.

（3）Qingshen granule combined with Western medicine basic therapy showed good clinical efficacy in improving symptoms, reducing syndrome scores, reducing urine protein and protecting kidney function in patients with chronic renal failure damp-heat syndrome.

第六节 材料与方法

1. 根据所给汉语提示完成句子。

（1）were purchased from; was obtained from

（2）after 3 months; every 3 weeks

（3）Anesthetized; as previously described

（4）was prescribed

（5）aged above 70; The proportion between male and female

2. 汉译英。

（1）Images were captured on days 1,3,5,7,9,11 and 13 and transferred to a personal computer for image analysis as described below.

（2）The treatment effect, as measured by the hazard ratio and its associated 95% confidence interval, was estimated with the use of the Cox proportional-hazards model.

（3）Patients with stable coronary artery disease were included in the study. A detailed description of the inclusion and exclusion criteria is included in the Supplementary Appendix. Patients who were eligible for the study underwent randomization after providing written informed consent.

（4）The mean age of 936 male patients was 48.5 years old (range 7–96); the mean age of 404 female patients was 49.6 years old (range 10–78).

（5）Sputum induction was performed according to the recommendations of the European Respiratory Society, and the samples were immediately processed with the use of dithioerythritol to separate cells from the fluid phase of sputum.

第七节 结果

1. 根据所给汉语提示完成句子。

（1）displays/shows/indicates/suggests; are due nearly entirely to

（2）respectively; a statistically significant but clinically small difference

（3）Treatment-emergent adverse events; The most frequently reported adverse reactions

（4）There were no significant effects

（5）accounted for; accounted for

2. 汉译英。

（1）After a median of 5 years of follow-up, the mean glycated hemoglobin level was lower in the intensive-control group (6.5%) than in the standard-control group (7.3%).

（2）At 6 to 8 weeks post partum, 552 women (75.3%) underwent a 75g oral glucose-tolerance test. In 62 of 270 women (23.0%) in the metformin group and 58 of 282 (20.6%) in the insulin group, glucose tolerance was impaired or diagnosed as diabetes.

（3）There was a statistically significant but clinically small difference in the mean gestational age at delivery between the metformin group (38.3 weeks) and the insulin group (38.5 weeks).

（4）Terbinafine was well tolerated. Side effects were mild to moderate in severity, and transient. The most common side effects were gastrointestinal symptoms (fullness, loss of appetite, nausea, mild abdominal pain, diarrhea) or nonserious forms of skin reactions (rash, urticaria).

（5）3 died of non-renal causes. 52% of the remaining 20 patients maintained stable renal function for at least 2 years. 4 of the 9 patients followed up for longer than 2 years had a relapse, but all responded again to therapy. No characteristic clinical symptoms prediction relapse were found, although nearly all had hematuria and proteinuria. Complications of therapy were frequent and might have contributed to death in 2 patients.

第八节 讨论

1. 用讨论的规范用语改写下列句子。

（1）In contrast to these results, Packer *et al*. reported that the RNA level of MUC13 was decreased in colon cancer.

（2）We obtained miRNA expression profiles of BCSCs, which provided a substantial basis for exploring the function of miRNAs in maintaining stem cell properties and the biological functions of BCSCs.

（3）In addition, we also detected the expression of some predicted miRNAs in the BCSCs.

（4）Excitingly, several AITD（autoimmune thyroid disease）susceptibility genes have been identified and characterized.

（5）To confirm that *DNMT3A* represses the expression of *Oct4* by altering the degree of DNA methylation, we analyzed the DNA methylation status in three key regions of *Oct4* by BGS.

（6）Rapid detection is the most prominent advantage of this method; as the sample detection step can be finished within 15 min.

2. 翻译下列句子。

（1）We reported a novel method

（2）suggesting a possible explanation for

（3）Some controversy exists regarding/as to

（4）Our findings support the hypothesis

（5）contrary to our hypothesis

（6）To our knowledge, this is the first study that demonstrates

（7）These results provide the experimental basis for

（8）these discrepancies are due to

第九节 结论

1. 把下列汉语句子翻译成英语。

（1）Examination of VEGF expression can help to select the patients who need chemotherapy and radiotherapy, and may be as an indicator of prognosis.

（2）Down-regulating TF expression and up-regulating TM expression of stimulated endothelial cells may be one of the mechanisms of GAG antithrombosis.

（3）These results are consistent with the use of buprenorphine as an acceptable treatment for opioid dependence in pregnant women.

2. 把下列英语段落翻译成汉语。

（1）妊娠期间出现的生理变化可提示机体出现慢性病的可能性。代谢综合征的典型变化亦可见于先兆子痫和妊娠期糖尿病，这些变化预示着机体将来有可能会发生心血管疾病和代谢性疾病。为此，临床上应抓住妊娠这个重要契机，对心血管疾病和代谢性疾病的危险因素进行筛查，提供相应的早期干预。

（2）本研究证明了复方中药制剂养血清脑颗粒通过抑制血管内皮细胞的紧密连接蛋白的降解、抑制质膜微囊-1 的表达改善缺血再灌注引起的脑水肿，进而改善脑梗死和神经元损伤，该结果提示养血清脑颗粒有可能成为应用于干预重度脑水肿的药物。

第十节　参考文献

以下内容摘自某医学专业论文的文献清单，请尝试以温哥华格式进行编排。

Blasi F. Atypical pathogens and respiratory tract infections. *European Respiratory Journal* 2004;55:23-5.

Burillo A, Bouza E. *Chlamydophila pneumoniae* infect. *Dis Clin North Am* 2010;10:72-4.

Ciarrocchi G, Benedetto F, Fogliani V, Magliano E, Del Prete R, Miragliotta G. Serological study on *Chlamydophila pneumoniae* in patients with community-acquired pneumonia. *New Microbiologica* 2004;9:26-8.

Garcia-Jardon M, Bhat VG, Blanco-Blanco E, Stepian A. Postmortem findings in HIV/AIDS patients in a tertiary care hospital in rural South Africa. *Tropical Doctor* 2010;2:11-3.

Kuo CC, Campbell LA. Chlamydial infections of the cardiovascular system. *Frontiers in Bioscience* 2003;12:34-8.

Lee SJ, Lee MG, Jeon MJ, *et al.* Atypical pathogens in adult patients admitted with community-acquired pneumonia in Korea. *Japanese Journal of Infectious Diseases* 2002;8:112-4.

Miyashita N, Obase Y, Fukuda M, Shoji H, Mouri K, Yagi S. Evaluation of serological tests detecting *Chlamydophila pneumoniae*-specific immunoglobulin M antibody. *Journal of Internal Medicine* 2006;23:112-5.

Miyashita N, Kawai Y, Yamaguchi T, *et al*. Evaluation of false positive reaction with ELISA for the detection of *Chlamydophila pneumoniae*-specific IgM antibody in adults. *Japanese Journal of Infectious Diseases* 2010;32:76-8.

Satpalhy G, Sharma A, Vasisht S. Immunocomb chlamydia bivalent assay to study chlamydia species specific antibodies in patients with coronary heart disease. *Indian Journal of Medical Research* 2005;7:53-5.

第三章　留学文书写作

2. 下面是一则个人陈述，请按照逻辑顺序重新排列段落。

（3）（2）（4）（1）（7）（5）（6）

下 篇

第二章 语法

1. 请为下列句子选择正确的动词形式。

（1）were　　　　（2）is　　　　（3）were　　　　（4）were

（5）is　　　　　（6）were　　　　（7）were was　　　（8）is

2. 请修改下列句子。

（1）The expression of *Oct4* in both Hela and Caski cells was also higher than <u>in</u> C-33A cells.

（2）Methodological comparison <u>showed</u> that the SPR biosensor <u>had</u> the same detection rate as traditional culture methods（*P*<0.05）.

（3）To determine functional role of YB1 in prostate cancer cell invasion,<u>we silenced YB1 gene expression in PC3 cells.</u>

（4）Hyland demonstrated that cervical cancers <u>contains</u> a subpopulation of stem-like cancer cells expressing Oct4 protein.

（5）The abnormal expression of miRNAs <u>may be involved</u> in human diseases,including cancer.

（6）In traditional Chinese medicine theory,Zheng,which <u>is</u> also called a syndrome or pattern, <u>is</u> the basic unit and a key concept.

（7）Figure 1 <u>shows</u> the amounts of pollution accumulated in China over the past two decades.

（8）The purpose of this article <u>is</u> to give the most direct answer possible to the direct question of how long advertising affects sales.

3. 请找出下列段落中的错误并改正。

Music,meditation and acupuncture are used to relieve stress. For those who have developed a dependency on tranquilizers,<u>acupuncture</u> is most effective,as long as <u>they</u> could get used to the needles.

4. 请用适当的动词时态填空。

（1）Table 2 graphically <u>represents</u> the change in ecological footprint and biocapacity over this period. As can be seen,an ecological deficit <u>emerged</u> in 1991 and <u>increased</u> dramatically in subsequent years. Although both biocapacity and ecological footprint <u>grew</u> gradually,the increase in the ecological footprint（2.5 fold）<u>was</u> much greater than the corresponding biocapacity（1.4 fold）. In 2006,the ecological deficit <u>reached</u> 1.05 gha,and the ecological footprint per capita <u>was</u> 2.11 gha compared with the biocapacity per capita of 1.06 gha. The consistent increase in the ecological footprint <u>can</u> be directly related to population growth and economic development. The ecosystems <u>have faced</u> the twofold impact of population growth coupled with an increasing per capita consumption rate.

（2）Over the past three decades,many researchers and engineers <u>have developed</u> several urban infrastructure designs to <u>meet</u> the dual needs of pavement stability and tree health. There <u>are</u> two fundamental approaches to these designs:engineered soils and suspended pavement.

Engineered soils <u>are</u> composed of course stone <u>mixed</u> with fine-textured mineral soil to create a high porosity matrix that <u>can</u> be compacted to engineering load-bearing standards yet <u>retain</u> physical properties conducive to aeration, hydration, and root elongation.

5. 请用适当的动词语态填空。

TCM-samples <u>were generated</u> by randomly combining herbs into 4-,5-,6-,7-,8-,9- and 10-herb recipes from a pool of 813 herbs with available information about their traditionally defined properties. These samples <u>were drawn</u> in such a way that they <u>were distributed</u> evenly in the sampling space. They <u>were checked</u> further to remove those that happen to be in the TCM+class. A total of 1,961 randomly assembled recipes <u>were selected</u> from this process to form the TCM-training set. The number of samples in the 4-,5-,6-,7-,8-,9- and 10-herb TCM-training set sub-groups are 501,251,211,267,231,290 and 210, respectively. A total of 5,039 randomly assembled recipes <u>were used</u> as the TCM-testing set. The number of samples in the 4-,5-,6-,7-,8-,9- and 10-herb TCM-testing set sub-groups are 499,749,789,733,769,710 and 790, respectively.

第三章 句法

1. 请分析下列句子属于哪种类型: simple sentence, compound sentence, complex sentence, compound-complex sentence。

　　(1) simple sentence　　　(2) complex sentence　　　(3) compound sentence

　　(4) complex sentence　　　(5) complex sentence　　　(6) compound-complex sentence

2. 请选择恰当的词或词组完成句子。

　　(1) In addition to　　　(2) Therefore, In contrast　　　(3) Consequently

　　(4) while　　　(5) Hence　　　(6) Furthermore

　　(7) because　　　(8) such as

3. 请根据句意重新排列下列句子的顺序。

　　(4)　(1)　(3)　(5)　(2)

4. 请找出下列句子中的错误并修改。

　　(1) Australian education centers will require a broad communication network, <u>and</u> inefficiencies will otherwise occur.

　　(2) Service costs to prospective students should be kept to a minimum educational fees <u>which</u> are already expensive.

　　(3) Using RT-PCR, <u>we</u> cloned and sequenced IL-12 p40c DNA from the RNA extracted from cord blood dentritic cells (DC) of newborns in Beijing, China.

　　(4) Notably, <u>neither ES cells nor iPS cells</u> had not been infected with a carcinogenic virus.

　　(5) The specificity analysis demonstrated that hybridization did not occur between nucleotide sequences with a single-base mismatch, which is partly consistent with <u>previous reports</u>. (Lorenzo *et al.*, 2008; Naiser *et al.*, 2008)

（6）The election campaign is in its final stages; two candidates remain.

（7）Blood pH was measured with a capillary electrode.

（8）Changes of the refraction angle as a result of nucleic acid hybirdization were recorded in real time and then converted to electrical signals. The signals were then converted to the concentration of analytes by the system software.

5. 请把下列句子中的汉语翻译成英语。

（1）As is shown   （2）may be related   （3）We compared

（4）significant differences   （5）It is well known that   （6）these similarities are due to

第四章　标点

请为下列句子添加标点。

（1）Conversely, abnormal social interactions are debilitating symptoms of several neuropsychiatric disorders, notably autism spectrum disorder（ASD）.

（2）To examine whether 5-HT release in the NAc shares these features, we performed two assays: real-time conditioned placed preference（CPP）and optogenetic intracranial self-stimulation.

（3）These behavioural effects of 5-HT in the NAc are markedly different from the acute reinforcing properties of the release of dopamine in the NAc, suggesting critical differences in the NAc circuitry modulation by which these major neuromodulators mediate their behavioural effects.

（4）"Adding or removing an ingredient sometimes doesn't much change the efficacy of a compound TCM prescription," says Kaixian Chen, president of the Shanghai University of Traditional Chinese Medicine.

（5）For example, strain M, which had been subjected to *in vivo* passaging and drug treatment, was the most genetically distinct; the 11 strains used by the connectivity map project 16 over a 10-year period clustered tightly together; and sibling strains D and E, which were only a few passages apart, were the closest to each other.

（6）The MCF7, HT29, MDAM453, and A375 cell lines were cultured in RPMI 1640.

（7）All strains of the same cell line were cultured under the same conditions, cell identity was confirmed, and the cells were confirmed to be mycoplasma-free.

（8）"There is obviously an essential difference between a TCM formula and other compound products," says Song. "The concept of fangyi is unique to TCM prescriptions and should be protected by the patent law."

（9）"There are millions of crocodiles in the world," Zain observes, "but only a few thousand tigers."

（10）The expression of 222 miRNA precursors was profiled in 32 commonly used cell lines of lung, breast, head and neck, colorectal, prostate, pancreatic, and hematopoietic cancers.

（陈涵静）